TO QUIT THIS CALLING

FIRSTHAND TALES

OF A

PEDIATRIC
PATHOLOGIST

All the best in 2006!
Gail Waldstein

To Quit This Calling

Firsthand Tales of a Pediatric Pathologist

GAIL WALDSTEIN, M.D.

G R p

Ghost Road Press
Denver, Colorado

Library of Congress Cataloging-in-Publication Data.
Waldstein, Gail, (1942—).
To Quit This Calling: Firsthand Tales of a Pediatric Pathologist
Ghost Road Press
ISBN 0977127222 (pbk.)
Library of Congress Control Number: 2005931453
Book and Cover Design: Sonya Unrein
Ghost Road Press

Denver, Colorado
ghostroadpress.com

Thanks to the editors of the following journals for first publishing these tales, some in slightly different versions, and to the contest judges who saw merit in my words:

To Quit This Calling (manuscript)
     The Bakeless: Finalist

"Oval Ovaries, Flowering Tubes: Another Infant Autopsy"
     New Letters: 1st, Reprinted *New Letters: The Literary Essays*; *Pushcart*: Nominated; NYC YMCA, 2nd

"All Kinds of Love"
     Asphodel; Writer's Digest: Honorable Mention

"The Internship"
     Women: A Journal of Liberation

"Because Life is Slippery"
     Alligator Juniper; Deep South Writers Conference: Honorable Mention; The Faulkner: 2nd

"Bandaged Archipelago"
     Arapahoe Community College Writer's Studio: Finalist; The Faulkner: Semi-Finalist

"ER Euphemism"
     Explorations 2000; Times of Sorrow, Times of Grace, Caduceus

"Madness: A Vivid Interior Void"
     Kaleidoscope; New Letters: Honorable Mention

"Lapse"
     Bayou

"Faith Forces"
     The MacGuffin; The Faulkner: Finaist; *Writer's West*: Finalist

"L.A. Territory"
     Palomar Showcase

"Weave"
     Bayou; Eugene Walter Contest:2nd

"Late Sentence"
     The Faulkner: Finalist

"Tremble
     Alligator Juniper; The Faulkner: Finalist

"The Date, The Rape & Dad"
     MadBlood

"Relish"
     The Faulkner: Semi Finalist

"Singing In the Ear Canal"
     Iowa Review: Finalist; *New Letters*: Finalist; *Writer's Digest* Honorable Mention; Faulkner: 2nd; Short Story Abroad: 3rd

"Ashes, Ashes"
     White Eagle Coffee Store Press: Honorable Mention

Thanks to all my writing teachers and to close women friends over the years who baby-sat, held both my hands through hard times, and love me despite myself: Fern, Susan, Daneen, Phyllis, Elizabeth, Lana, Louise, Jinny, Julie, Margaret, and Hildegard. I am honored by those who read for me beyond the bonds of friendship, intelligently and with deep care, Connie, Erin, and Pam.

I owe my medical education to the Robert Wood Johnson Foundation scholarship. I am grateful for support from the Rocky Mountain Women's Institute; the Colorado Council for the Arts, and the Helene Wurlitzer Foundation. Special thanks to Sonya and Matt, who believe in me and birthed this.

for my children Sarah, Samantha and Saul
for their gifts of life, laughter, and love

Oval Ovaries, Flowering Tubes:
Another Infant Autopsy   12

All Kinds of Love   20

An Internship (1968)   24

Because Life is Slippery   33

Bandaged Archipelago   45

ER Euphemism   60

Madness: A Vivid Interior Void   62

Lapse   72

Faith Forces   80

L.A. Territory   94

Weave   100

Relish   113

Late Sentence   136

Tremble   140

The Date, The Rape & Dad   161

Ashes, Ashes   185

Singing in the Ear Canal   219

I am not what I am. I am what I do with my hands.

—Louise Bougeois

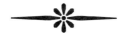

The thing about working in a children's hospital is, you open the huge entrance door first thing in the morning, somedays it's so heavy you need both hands to pull it out, it opens out for safety, but the thing is, you could have had a bad night: diarrhea, bronchitis, a child up with fever and an earache. Or a fight with your husband, hard enough to stop your heart, word-hurling-horrid, a final loveless loss. Your parents could be sick; you could be early in a pregnancy you're scared about; or later, estranged from a child...but you pull open that door and walk into the land of sick children, sick and dying, and there's laughter. Bald kids in wagons with chemo drips on the side, sucking a lolly. Children with bandages on their heads so huge, you think whale-headache. Teens missing a limb, or with steel rods in their backs, straightening a curve. Blue-lipped babies that need a new heart. And your problem, whatever issue broke the day, narrows to a line, a dot, an irrelevancy, and you snap your fingers, fling that worry away.

Oval Ovaries, Flowering Tubes
Another Infant Autopsy

The Children's Hospital, Denver, 1990.

Holding a scalpel's second nature for me, and when I clasp the stainless handle, it is *my* instrument, in the way a writer owns her pen, or a priest holds the host. There is faint blood loss. I pull the pliable, fragile skin toward her face, gripping it taut with toothed forceps, while I scissor dissect with my right hand. Precise pressure's imperative, too little and the child's chest will not free of its flesh, too much and it will rip and tear. This fiercely physical process is only possible if my diener and friend, Fern, trades morgue jokes with me. We flip through family updates, everyday talk, politics, the weather, and later, much, much later, we share intimate, secret sexual encounters, real or imagined. Bad days, with five autopsies, we dip into pornographic fantasies. Any conversation is appropriate if it bridges this chasm of unthinkability. We are examining a child's corpse, dissecting and sampling someone's beloved baby.

This is the sixty-seventh this year; it's barely the end of May. I remember earlier days, when I was fresh in my career. Almost thirty years ago, vegetarianism wasn't popular or politically correct. Even back then, I ate only salads and eggs for weeks at a time, avoiding red meat, its stringy, grained consistency and the way it smelled cooking, like the fried char of organs when I seared them with a red-hot spatula blade to obtain sterile cultures. I no longer owned a ravenous appetite. The salivation meat had once evoked in me was closer to the way spit pools preceding nausea. I sampled infants' lungs, heart-blood, spinal fluid to document infection, to identify the species of bacteria or fungus. Viral identification was impossible in the '60s and early '70s. In those days queasiness rippled through me when someone at an adjacent cafeteria table ate a hamburger. This revulsion grew so strong that even dinning out with my first husband was abbreviated, ephemeral as an affair.

A quick abdominal incision now, straight down the midline. I stop at the pubis. The examination begins in earnest. Fern records measurements as I shout them out, how far the liver and spleen jut below the diaphragm, the length of the small bowel, how long its insertion. How it's rotated in this belly. Routines and numbers numb us both.

I remember when focus was very difficult. Speed, facility, certainty were not yet in me, the habit of autopsy something I didn't deliberately plan. Fern breaks my reverie with, "Did you hear the one about Bill and Hillary riding into the hills of West Virginia for an outing, right before his inauguration?" She's distancing herself today; her granddaughter's precisely this infant's age.

"No, I haven't heard that one. Go on."

"Over in the backwoods there, in some hollow of an Allegheny valley, well they're riding along and..."

I test the chest for air, plunge a large bore needle between the ribs. The plunger does not yield: there is no pneumothorax, no free air in the chest. A sudden blowout of an emphysematous bleb did not suddenly kill this previously healthy baby.

Now I cover her face with the skin flap from her chest. This will hide her staring eyes, spare her, spare us.

With heavy bone scissors, I clip each rib in the central, cartilaginous area. I need two hands these days to close the bone scissors, my loss of hand strength's annoying and new, but I don't ask even Fern for help. I regrasp my favorite blunt tipped scissors, dissect the chest plate, her sternum, from the pericardial surface. My hand-scissors expose her heart, lungs, thymus, pleural cavities. Chest symmetry is imperfect because the heart lies almost entirely in the left hemithorax. The pink, plump thymus is riddled with blood-red dots, petechia. The billowy salmon lungs are similarly studded. They show full expansion: gasp-like reality. Rib imprints delicately dent their surfaces, like rungs of a ladder.

As I get the lung culture, a minute amount of clear fluid accumulates on the cut surface, frothy bubbles cling to the scalpel edge, as if it still contained breath, her final drowning cry.

Somedays, I see my years in pediatric pathology as one long contusion, a bruise of anger at God for permitting diseases to attack little children. And while there are moments, hours at a stretch, that I'll get lost in a baby's body, dissecting tissue planes delicately, identifying anomalies or variations of normal, locating the blood supply for a tumor, the thrombus in a vessel thin as thread, there's always, always the knowledge that the parents' grief will never end—no matter what I find. And it's not that I don't love the excitement of frozen sections, snap freezing tissue, immediately calling, benign or malignant, informing the surgeon how to proceed. That's high drama, and like all adrenaline junk, it's its own kind of reward. It's just that too many days, I can't tell them what they want to hear, that the tumor is benign, or their margins, free.

The heart. I need my reading glasses now, and strong, concentrated light. I remove the thymus from the straining engorged vessels, pale blue and white. A nick will obscure the field in blood, contaminate culture results, crimp time for my conference preparation, which is thin. For this part of the dissection, I choose minuscule scissors. The great veins from above and below enter the right atrium as expected. The pulmonary veins, thick, short, and navy-blue, enter the stubby left atrium, with its weird scythe-shaped extension. All is in order. The left side of the heart is hidden in babies, immediately behind the right ventricle. This one is properly positioned, posterior, normal. It is firm and thick and pink. The anterior, right ventricle looks as if two white arteries arise from its flat top. Gentle small scissoring of the wispy tissue reveals the pulmonary trunk is up front and slightly to the right. It connects to the aorta by a long winding ductus. Closed now, of course. The baby is, was, three months old.

The aorta does arise from the left and posterior chamber, arches gracefully into the left hemithorax, branches appropriately.

I use the back of my gloved hand to readjust my glasses and push back a strand of graying hair from my cheek. I check the clock, enough time to gather myself and the slides. I recall when a single post mortem would slog through three-quarters of a day, accompanied by a vague sinking feeling, somewhere between hunger and bandaged fatigue. My mind would glaze over those afternoons as though I'd gorged on an ice cream sundae. I was not nimble, had a beginner's stuttering technique, history now, belonging to a woman I've lost.

I don't hesitate or ever apply uneven pressure in my slicing now. I no longer make ratchety lines, surface chatter which exposes an amateur's hand. Or, one who doesn't care enough about her tools to keep them sharp, isn't sufficiently finger-informed to use the right force on each organ, whose liquid/gaseous/solid structure demands individualized tension. I'm good.

Back then I was conflicted too, disturbed by the dichotomy, being a woman and doing profane, shunned, prohibited work. The severe isolation and steel echoes of the morgue shrouded me like a family secret, married in a way, to these death-cloaked children. The choking anathema of uncleanness, reminiscences of menstrual huts, old Hebrew prohibitions, untouchability, haunted me. Shamed among my colleagues who practiced living medicine. Practice, practice until they got it right. Or sent me their mistakes. I grew a carapace of glib expertise.

"Well, see, it was this beautiful sunny day and they were running low on gas, so Bill pulled into a station." I know she's superstitiously protecting her grandchild.

Part of what slowed me early was the ineluctable death of a child. That abyss of no sense, no meaning. I was more distractible too, because my own children were small, and needful. They called me every day after school, every single day. There was also my guilt, for having made it to adulthood. And the way I prayed in the morgue, a sort of God-bargain: that if I performed this autopsy with dedication and focus, a sort of penance, my own children would remain safe. And healthy.

I visually inspect the warm, wet, pink-white intestines. They are where they belong, neither twisted nor infarcted. The liver is brick red and dominates the abdominal cavity. It weighs the anticipated number of grams. The spleen, high in the left upper abdomen, is soft, purple, with a wrinkled gray capsule. The stomach, white with morning milk curds, befouls the air as it's opened. The acidic scent moves me with a purpose. I still have to organize my slides. I remove the snake of intestines with blunt-tipped, curved scissors, angled at exactly thirty degrees between bowel wall and slick mesentery. The rope coils through my gloved fingers with the precision of a finely oiled machine. My movements are as smooth and automatic as the melt of an ice cream cone when scorched by the tongue-tip of a city child, late August.

The pelvis dips deep and dark, holds an empty fibrous bladder and a pink, evacuated rectum. Positioned between these organs are two tiny, gleaming white oval ovaries, attached to wisps of tubes with flower-like ends, forever useless. The tentacles at the ends of the Fallopian tubes always remind me of sea anemones. It's a problem in bars with fish tanks. As I remove the intra-abdominal contents I come to the fixed organs, sewed into the retroperitoneal space by gauzed, translucent tissue planes. Here are paired gold, triangular adrenals, nested symmetrically on top of smooth tan kidneys. After removal I slice each organ at one centimeter intervals with a blade sharp as a spinster's tongue. I examine the stacked slices for clues, lesions, the tiniest disturbance. I see no abnormalities.

I prefer babies because of my sensitivities...their organs rarely smell, the body is compact, and the head can be opened with thick scissors. I do not have to resort to the piercing, shrill shriek of the bone saw. Its vibrations are so terrible they penetrate my arms and tremble my fingers with an electric dance that vibrates hours after I've left the morgue.

The cranium. Most consider it sacred. I enter this perfectly round, golden-curled head and find a deeply furrowed, soft brain. Encased by thick, gray-green scum. Meningitis. Unsuspected. This will have huge physician and parental repercussions. It will necessitate many conferences, much counseling. Medico-legal issues will be raised. This type of disease rarely sneaks up. There *are* signs, and symptoms. Fever. Nausea. Irritability. Convulsions. Vomiting. Apathy. I will have to bear witness. Speak with the parents. Perhaps even hold the hands of the healer, who may have missed the diagnosis.

Still, this is more satisfying than the baby who dies of SIDS. The explosion of sudden, unexpected, forever unexplained infant death. An appalling vacuum of no answer. The terminal burden that rings across parents' lifetimes: the silence of gray. The never ending *Why?* And my inadequate, *I don't know.*

I unglove, the beginning taste of a small satisfaction, an answer, moves the corners of my mouth up, ever so slightly.

"Okay, lady, it's a wrap. We'll do the leukemic at one-thirty sharp. Right after lunch. You can finish the Billary story then."

As I walk the long corridor to my plant-embraced office with its wide windows, I anticipate the sunshine, even for a few minutes. I think how infrequently now I really need a microscope for autopsies. I have reached that stride that approaches the reputations of my nineteenth century predecessors, Virchow, Rokitansy. They could diagnose anything by gross examination alone. Imagine a mere woman doing their esteemed work. They would rotate in their graves.

"I do this," I tell my few non-medical friends in a well rehearsed litany, "to educate physicians. Show them where they went wrong. To determine the effectiveness of therapy, whether it was appropriate, and sufficient. If their diagnoses were accurate."

When I was young and glib, I would quip, "I have to have the last word."

But I am weighted with my job now. I know the somber information I must gather to tell the family with great accuracy if their next child, or a subsequent pregnancy would, might, will, come to such a gruesome, premature end.

I call the pediatrician who cared for this infant to tell him the news. While I'm on hold, I arrange the slides chronologically to recount a story of a different child's death. I place figures in the slide tray, then gross photos, microscopic pictures, and finally, the subcellular details in black and white electron microscopy. I blink away the gray-green crust of infected meninges around this morning's brain, pulsing at the periphery of my vision. When the doctor finally gets on the line, I am guarded as I describe the degree of meningitis. His voice cracks on *Thank you*.

I take a deep breath and smell the stale fish-tank odor of that particular organism, Klebsiella, as I replace the phone. I collect my notes, grab the slide tray, my purse and leave the cradling noontime sun.

As I approach the lectern I notice the young, eager, unformed faces in the audience. All these children really, posing as interns, residents, house staff. I have deep tongue-kissed death so often, I no longer shudder, grimace, or even wince. I suck formaldehyde perfume into my lungs daily, like an elixir, and still emerge each evening from the hospital like a human being, like clockwork. I palpate death's interior through my scissored and knifed hands so often, I sometimes think I own some skill for excising pain. I honestly believe I'll continue to handle this for years.

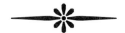

As a child on the lower east side, my grand-mother was always investigating, overly curious. One day she stuck her hand into her mother's wringer, on the back of the washing machine. Her mother cleaned houses and did laundry for New York's wealthy. It was the turn of the century, with all those romantic ideals for women, so that even in her eighties, if Nana said something off-color, she'd hide her wrinkled face behind her hands, like a coquette. The stub end of her middle finger had a curled nail like a crochet hook, and it stood as warning, to be cautious, not to be so inquisitive.

I believe genetics is stronger than a mere wife's tale.

I could never tell my mother about Susannah. And what she lets the boys do. I keep seeing her breasts stick straight out from her chest, the soft way her hair curls around her neck. How when she laughs, her hair slides over the top of those breasts and stops, just before they meet, in that crease-place in the center. The space where other girls wear a cross.

I don't have breasts like that. Neither does my mother. They don't run large in my family. In the middle of my chest is a medal of St. Jude. Mother gave me that for my first holy communion. She said he's the saint of the impossible. Mom wears a medal too, a turquoise one of the Virgin. The blue matches her eyes. It's the first thing she fists when something goes wrong, when someone surprises her, or hurts her too much. Like when Dad gets really mean and hits one of us, or starts his attack, the shouting and throwing things, and then the wheezing that takes him into the hospital.

I hope hanging around Susannah means I'll grow those kinds of breasts one day, because then the boys will see me. Now I'm just a tag-along. I help her with her homework, even though she's a grade ahead of me. And if she has to go to the store to buy supper, she lets me come.

Last week we went behind the building and fooled around with some boys. They were from Rahway, and there were needles on the ground and a strange smell, a little like Dad's medicine. They were loud and dreamy looking, and later she said they were shooting up. I don't know what that means exactly, but it must be important, because Susannah never gives orders, but she did make me swear I wouldn't tell anybody about it. I would never squeal anyway.

Three days a week I get to go home with her. Her mom works.

Susannah has very pale skin and some days she takes some of her mother's cream and puts little pats on her chin and forehead and cheeks. And then soothes it in. Last Wednesday she put some on my face, cool and slippery and smelling like apricots. She didn't seem to mind touching those three ugly pimples on my forehead.

I love to watch her practice her face in the mirror. She arches her black eyebrows, waves her eyelids, spreads her lips and studies her teeth. They're very white and small and even. Then she presses the sides of her mouth toward the center. She tries sad, frightened, angry, surprised, as different faces. She says she's going to grow up and be an actress. I think she's trying on poses for the boys. She says she's leaving when she turns sixteen, and I believe her. My mother saw her one day after school and said Susannah was bad, that she dressed like a slut, that I shouldn't hang around with her. She said, "Mark my words, that one will grow up to be a whore."

I tell Mom that I've been chosen to stay and wash blackboards, help the teacher change decorations, clap erasers, because I'm such a good student. And I am a good student. I can't tell her I go to Susannah's. I don't tell her how every Friday, we steal two cigarettes from her father's pack on his side of the bed. Or about the first time I took a drag and got so sick and dizzy. I thought God or one of those saints was coming for me. Not for the cigarettes you know, but for the lies. It felt like I'd never be able to breathe again without that fire shooting down into my chest. And because of that, I wondered if I'd have breathing trouble, like my father. I sucked hard for air, I think I even wheezed a little. I wondered if I did get asthma, if Mom would love me the way she does him.

It's years and years later, and I'm at a high school reunion when someone asks about Susannah. All our parents are dead now, and it no longer matters whether Mother loved me enough. Or if she felt cheated because I censored so much of my growing up from her. I have adult children of my own who funneled through experiments with drugs. We discuss these adolescent secrets over Thanksgiving desserts, but only after a lot of wine. Their confessions leave me vertiginous and breathless, and I understand that ignorance isn't the worst sin. Heroin's recycled back, hip again, along with black leather, slick hair, motorcycles.

It's our thirtieth high school reunion, the boys are men, stout and bald, the girls still sexy, but strong and savvy too. Not everyone returns of course. Someone mentions Susannah, says she left New Jersey, moved to a border town, Nogales, Tijuana, somewhere out West, with ranches and cowboys. Then they quickly cut their eyes and whisper, "She owns her own business, sells love and forgiveness."

I see her as she will always be for me, slender shoulders crossed by satin straps, her special bra, the one she modeled for me that last afternoon before I got caught. It was her dating bra, salmon colored, with a slim line of lace at the top of each cup. I close my eyes as a classmate dances me around the floor, and try not to look at his neck. It's hers I'm avoiding, with its purple vein at the base, pulsing as she flings her head back, abandons herself to laughter. Her airiness hypnotizes me again, as if this were last Sunday, right after sock-hop. *Look*, she says, *how silly the boys are, white shirts, navy trousers with skinny belts, and ties. Not one of them knows enough to wear suede shoes.* She whispers this against my neck, her breath hot and graveled, years of smoke.

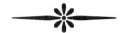

Nana taught me to crochet when I was seven. She pulled me on her lap, skinny legs dangled over old, swollen knees. Her hands were sure and huge and soft above mine. She looped multicolored cord around my left pinkie, then circled my index finger, which had to stay upright, taut against the pull of the thread, to keep the stitches even. She clasped my right hand below hers, twirled the crotchet hook, leading my wrist in a semicircle, and slipped red or bright green through the loop of indigo, forming a chain from thread, togetherness, and thin air.

Nana taught me after supper, full and relaxed, I leaned into her strength and safety.

As I grew, I loved making things for others, like Nana. I embroidered violet peace symbols and snow-white peace doves on denim shirts for my husband. Hand crocheted sweaters, and hand-sewed dresses for my daughters. New blue baby blankets, a jacket and cap for my son.

Grumble. I fly to Denver alone, very pregnant with our first baby, mid-June. I have gestational diabetes, and a handsome husband who won a fellowship in immunology here. He will drive cross country in a few days, join me. I have never known such loneliness and fear. I sleep on a rollaway rental bed in an empty apartment, read pages of orientation and the hospital manual each night by flashlight. I walk ten blocks to and from the hospital, begin my training. I'm a pediatric intern, also a patient, cared for by the obstetric service and an endocrinologist.

I make it through June and July, although too many nights I'm late at the hospital, eleven p.m., when I should've been home by six. I have feet so swollen I'm unbalanced walking, my legs ache, and many days my hands are clumsy, boggy. I'm chronically exhausted. At home I still cleave to Camelot, do the dishes after dinner, silently damn anti-dishwasher ecologists.

"Dr. Rosen, Dr. R."

"Core zero, Ward B!" Mid-lunch, my intern partner and I run up three flights, panting, he beats me by a minute. It's the blue-black baby with an incurable disease; all his nerve cells accumulate lipids which should break down and be excreted. He has almost no brain function, does not respond to any stimuli. A squalid, limp infant who suddenly, one day, smiled, then resumed gagging, drooling. His parents are devastated, and broke. This is a time of weighing my patients' health against my own. This is a year of dwindling sanity, and bitter, brief, power: addictive and depleting. Only interns are allowed to write orders for the patients on the pediatric wards. Consultants and residents and attendings can write notes, but I alone decide which tests can be performed, what medications given, their doses, and when, or if, the child should have surgery. Only the intern. It's a great way to learn, instant responsibility. But I wonder if the parents understand the recklessness, the terrible vulnerability of their children.

There's an incessant gnawing fear of losing grip, of slashing through routines, of making mistakes, of killing children. We all double check our math calculating drug doses, worry about fuck-ups in judgment; we're all sleep-deprived stupid. I always feel like I'm right on the verge of screaming, for someone, for help, for someone to hold my hand, which must caress, comfort, calm. Where's the aseptic perfection, the clarity I believed would come with the white coat?

I long for the oblivion of medical school, the semi-aware student, passively watching, passing judgment on the judges. Senior year I actually registered to vote as a "housewife" because my scholarship wouldn't have covered tuition if my legal residence were still New Jersey with my parents. Temple had become a state school that year. The housewife role was partially true, I wasn't working for money. My husband was a resident then, earning twice his internship salary, almost three thousand a year. It doesn't matter if it was 1967, that income still left us eligible for food stamps. Only neither of us had time to get them. Besides, I did all the tidying up, made meals, took laundry to the Laundromat, fed his friends, loved him the nights I could.

As an intern, the need for free time gets buried below motherhood, doctorhood, being a wife, desire pulsing occasionally, but so deeply and infrequently, I no longer know what's going on inside.

Air, fresh air, I need to breathe. My belly grows, presses my diaphragm, constricts my lungs.

Orientation. They whiz us through a maze: wards, stairs, water fountains, plush, carpeted treasure room of—books, the medical library. Photo ID, snap. Little conversation, too much teasing by my soon-to-be-partners about my belly. My hesitant globular gait, a waddle, reinforces my embarrassment.

But why? A wife's more radiant pregnant, so why does a strange woman appear grotesque, obscene, particularly in a professional—a man's—world? She's still the same head, face, breasts as when she's menstruating. Only now the reaction is close to contempt, a cultural taboo. Or maybe it's this physical evidence of passion, my belly, the men are afraid of. Could medicine men fear sexuality? Why all the snickers?

Child delivered.

Beautiful, normal, normal, normal, normal girl. Tears of happiness. Laughter at fear dispelled, agony screams passed. The tiny wonder, red-pink, sucks, grows, smiles. My husband is not saddened by a girl. Double relief. Wonderful, tired happy days at home with babe. Has anyone given birth before?

Furtively, early September, I wheel baby Tori, *turtledove*, to the hospital to get my paycheck. They have given me two weeks vacation and I take two more weeks as sick leave. I do not want to go back to work. I go to quell my husband's nagging. I fear recognition in the halls, being scolded to return—to watch children die. I sneak in to avoid being bullied by staff, fellows, residents, students. Who is lower than the intern?

Then the terrible task of finding a surrogate mother for Tori. Love-child must have love. I conquer my gnawing want, the need to be necessary, the fleeting, willful desire to choose a cold sitter so my baby's smile will sunny only my short hours at home. If only altruism spontaneously generated. Wretched interviews, nauseated days, frantic, tear-stained nights. A lady with much affection comes.

Return...thinking I should return...home. Always, always knowing neither arena has all of me. My husband, quietly supportive, undemanding. But nudging me to work, to the world. My babygirl, playful, a pink fluff of squeals, screams, delights. What I recall now of her first year is fatigue and guilt.

But there are medical compensations: I rescue a young boy, three years old, wrecked by Salmonella. He vomits blood, has constant bloody diarrhea, his eyes are sunken in a faded, terrible face. A shriveled shell of a boy—I pull him through. I hand-pump bags of saline and blood, and antibiotics the whole night.

And there are the beaters. My rage at children's fractured bones, ambivalent adult emotion, is not hidden; in this domain I'm unprofessional. I want to murder these parents. I want to take home the contorted, confused children. But they cling, with wiry, bruised limbs, like tentacles suckering strong, to these same parents. This *is* love, they've been told, and it curls inside them like a wire-spring, trust and belief.

There are nights plating cultures, sipping coffee at one a.m., curved over a microscope, avoiding the suffering parents. The remnants of my humanity shred when leukemia must be discussed. The incomprehension in the eyes of the parents, they never hear anything after I say, malignant. The piercing stare of the seven-year-old who enters our lie that he is excited about returning home to his brothers, his pony. He knows. I cannot swallow solid food for a week. I slam open the exit door to the stairwell, sit on the cold cement, and weep. His large, puffy eyes, and immaculate white skin follow me everywhere. In the car, in the on-call room, in my bedroom, when I hold my daughter. His angel-drawing hangs over sink-space; he inhabits my home, haunts my days with his stoic laughter.

The fifteen-year-old beauty hospitalized with a "blood disease" during a brash TV-leukemia-education week. Sedated, she burbles her diagnosis, her death, things she will not admit awake, either to herself or her parents. There's safety in denial, maybe a kind of grace even.

I thread a bitter, shallow, tenuous relationship with Spanish-American parents of an eighteen year old boy/man. The family's devout, encased in multiplying superstitions as death nears. Can we save him, *por favor*. He's unconscious, suffocating, dying. *¿Que?* How do I answer?

Can I wield the morphine-laden needle? Will I be intact or Lady Macbeth stained after the injection? Pros and cons churn: my own early Catholicism, my conversion to ethical Judaism. A noted hematologist, Noble Staff Doctor, says, *He's been my patient for three years*, swallows. *Yes, I'd give him more morphine.* Then the doctor goes home.

The tear-drawn Mother watching her flesh suffer, begging: *No more pain. No more experiments, no death, no.*

The boy/man, seeing sometimes, sleeping most days. Dark eyes beg for life, nostrils flare, men's hands crawl up my arm. Does a god will this? Can a human participate; never mind my eyes are lowered, shoulders stooped, heart and spine shiver. Dare one only watch?

The injection backfires. Morphine has a side effect I do not know: it dilates pulmonary arteries so the young man gets more oxygen, survives, struggling, but no longer blue, for another full week.

Not everything is ick. Some sick children improve. *Dr. Rosen, don't wear your hair up. You look so pretty with it down. Can I hold your baby Dr. Rosen?* Snuggles, winks.

Tomorrow Jancie, you go home. She giggles her thanks.

As an intern I ride ambulances, sirens screech, while out the back window, dawn fingers a navy sky. One midnight a vulgar ambulance assistant runs a hand under my skirt. Repulsive ass. I adjust the incubator temperature and oxygen, watch the baby struggle for life, do not acknowledge his stealth move, or his hand's withdrawal. Yet somehow, this touch is more human than all the sophisticated, semi-verbal propositions of my white-clad, professional colleagues.

Infants in incubators: amphibians. Wrinkled prunes pried from death by gadgets which chart temperature, intake, hand-twitch cycles. Another alarm, another no-sleep night. Spinal taps, respirator care, minuscule, thread-fine veins suck in drugs, food, life.

A triumph of sorts: I deny resuscitation to a large-headed, paralytic baby with spinal lumps and roll-back eyes. The parents want, beg, sign orders for DNR, DO NOT

RESUSCITATE, but the cardiac surgery fellows want the baby's heart, want him kept alive until they have a recipient. He dies on my watch, two a.m., in my arms.

A week later I begin intrathecal tetracycline, a forbidden drug in newborns because it stains teeth, may incorporate into bone. I insert the catheter into his spinal canal, squirt in the first dose, alone in his isolation room. Conventional drugs have failed three times in this two month old preemie. He has a resistant strain of E. Coli meningitis. Fellows, residents, other interns, spit warnings: there are protocols. They clasp trembling hands the afternoon the department chair approaches, on rounds. Two breeches: a direct, non chain-of-command approach (I speak directly to the chairman) and recommend the unmentionable drug. His okay's given. *When will you begin therapy?*

I started it two hours ago, sir.

Weeks of no sleep show up one shadowy Sunday, supermarketing. My daughter's happy, cookie-munching, and the cart is filled when I add two cans of Hunt's tomato paste for spaghetti sauce. It's April, the redbud's in bloom, but suddenly my husband takes the cans out, puts in generic.

No, the taste is different, I say, *it won't work.*

No, he says. *The Hunt brothers support the war.* The afternoon turns sullen. I leave the cart, the groceries, the store, reality, carry my frightened baby into the sun. I say I need the mountains—I am shaking uncontrollably. My daughter screams; I cry. My husband follows, paralyzed, waits for insanity to leave. What I really need is sleep, weeks and weeks of sleep, and food. But that will not come for more than a year.

There are other times, chirping spring days, hectic, bustling hours in the hospital, when I forget I have a home, a child, I am so busy. One May day I'm late to clinic and tongue-lashed by a very tall professor. He screams, *Irresponsible,* at top volume in front of parents, patients, in the crowded waiting room. Empty fart-head. I touch his lapel, *Please let's go to your office. Let me explain;* I hear the catch in my voice. But no. He continues, *Who do you think you are, someone extraordinary, Dr. Rosen?* I stomp by the raving man, mutter, calculating my pitch and volume, *Stuff it up your ass.*

Ashamed, triumphant, I am brought down by one more indiscretion. Reprimands and rumors speckled my entire year; this is a small, closeted world.

The first was a grotesque, lurid fanny-pat, on rounds, right after I returned from having my baby. A staff man, whose ego ate his judgment, when this kind of behavior was condoned. Of course, everyone in authority was male then. I bided my time. One sunny Friday afternoon this same professor waxed into a long, complex, and incorrect, description of the Rh factor; how it initiates antibody formation in the mother against the fetus. I let him continue, in front of a grand-rounds audience. When he finished, I corrected him, out loud. My father-in-law discovered the Rh factor. Large ego injured, large payment extracted. The house-staff director called me within an hour, *Your attitude, my dear, is not self-deprecating enough.*

I told my side, and the director laughed until he wiped tears from his eyes, advised being sweeter, deferential, *You do know what the word means.*

I'm called back again, bawled out for incompetence, for insufficient knowledge, for inadequate skill? No. For lack of respect.

Who's my accuser? Oh, we can't tell you, because last time you betrayed our confidence. You went back and confronted the gentleman, made him apologize for brushing against you, an accident, while you humiliated him in public.

Well, he should get his facts straight if he's teaching grand-rounds.

Anyway, your attitude's bad for the esprit de corps.

What are you talking about?

You question the value of night call, every other night. You've made remarks as to whether lack of sleep could impair judgment. My dear, we've run this program for decades. We turn out superlative pediatricians, top drawer.

I chew on this for a few days, arrive at the chief resident. A major misogynist, who hated medical women, usurping, white frocked broads, because one of them beat his college chum out of an admission to medical school, a "she." My being a Jewess, an Easterner, doesn't help.

On the rug for strike three, telling the tall bully to stuff it, exploding in the reception area like that, I expect I'll get canned. But no, I must silence all responses for the last month and a half of internship. I barter honest expression for completion. The machine, oiled with smiles and whimpering yesses, wins. I know something terrible will happen to me because of insincere compliance. I just don't know where or when.

Fire me, I offered. But three other interns had quit by then. They needed warm bodies.

And the housestaff director knew my residency was to be in pathology. *Perhaps we can accommodate a few idiosyncrasies longer.*

I'm already pregnant with my second baby as the year ends. I'm superstitiously careful about many things; I walked two blocks outside the hospital building in Philadelphia with my first pregnancy to avoid the radiology department. Now I take identical precautions with this pregnancy. To accompany a baby for cardiac catheterization, I drape four lead aprons over myself, almost kneeling from the weight, but my entire torso is guarded from scatter. I hand off patients who have infections that might cause intrauterine damage to my intern partners, men who by now love and care for me—we've worked long trenched nights for a year, no sleep, bad food; we are life-bonded.

My husband is deep in his research, brings experiments home to the top refrigerator shelf at least once a week. He teaches himself guitar, buys a Martin. He's active in anti-war protests. We move to a rental house whose attic stores turn-of-the-century books, on phrenology, racial profiling. We are mesmerized to read scientific defenses, tables, graphs. I'll be home nights now, will cook suppers. My husband gives me Julia Child's first book for my birthday. I'll be able to rock my daughter to sleep every night. She is strong and curious and so, so beautiful.

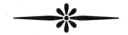

During my internship, my stomach was always queasy after an on-call, sleepless night. I brought bagels or wheat toast to morning rounds and sneak-ate as interns presented new admissions, complicated cases. Attendings commented, often humiliating the presenter with wisdom and experience. This was 1969, physicians still smoked; our chairman sucked cigars, every single morning. The chief resident called me into a stairwell one day, his index finger half an inch from my face, "No food at rounds. It distracts from the importance, like you don't take things seriously."

"I'll stop eating if he'll stop blowing his goddamned cigar smoke in my face." I'd learned by then that women were only heard if they used aggressive tones and foul language. The main man never lit up in the room again, but he always held a stub cigar between two fingers, like a dare.

Because Life is Slippery

Colorado General Hospital, August, 1968.

Hard. Sweat drenching hard. Difficult enough to be memory destroying, that hard. And stone dense.

Labor is not frivolously named. The perfect roundness of me betrays the unequal-to-the-task way I feel. Pregnant. Weighted. It bites me in two. Will I be able to love him and the new baby? Will it be normal? Will I?

It should be granite, it's that hard.

A bone ball, my belly with our love's labor, knots me. The roundness hardens, bears down, and I hang over the smooth marble, fetoid, praying for release.

I breathe again as it shrieks into my bladder, low, and steady. It rummages my anterior abdomen, above my joy, fire in the slick, stretched underside, a place that's been invisible for months. A hurricane of pain, increasingly unbearable.

"Don't push down yet, dear. This isn't hard labor." The nurse, book-informed, insists that it will not hurt until it gets to my back.

"When your spine begins to rip, *that* is labor."

She prattles knowledge, peddles faux pity. Later she panders pain meds.

My labor never goes to my back. Not with this, my first birth, nor with the second, labor-intense infant. Not even with the third. It's always razorsharp, frazzling, up-front. How I live my life, and where I wear my maternities. They never spread my hips. Progesterone pumps pontoon, Rubenesque breasts, long before the baby. They almost balance my belly, a circular ledge, bugling with new. I rest my arms on this curved shelf, crossed in purpose.

Part of me wants to be pampered, to be a lady in waiting, sprawl on a chaise lounge, contemplative, in velvets and lace. This is my first baby; it's still a time of residue: Kennedy's Camelot. I'm so ecstatic in my pregnancy I wear maternity dresses long before the slightest protrusion. I flaunt my fecundity before fellow students.

Another part of me knows that pampered femininity's racing toward extinction. Dylan's *the times, they are a changin'* is happening: now.

Senior year in medical school my interior schism begins. I am manacled to patients, crushing schedules, bedpans. My desire to help humanity, to live with excitement and challenge, and the ignorance of youth, lets me spend myself wildly. The fainting couch sentiment, the seductress-femme Mother tried to inculcate, has a skirted appeal. At home, when my husband's on call, I cry, get abysmally lonely late-nights, crave protection.

When I'm on call, I sweat through long, stanched nights, haul huge bleeding bodies from rusting carcasses of city ambulances. I gag around gurneys, then adjust my posture, reel patients through hallways, into bespattered emergency operating rooms. There's the Philadelphia Saturday night specials: a mucoid mix of alcohol, half-digested dinner, and bile that spews through raging lips and spread nostrils. I learn disease in my pores.

And like every doctor, this process of learning devours acres of humanity. Empathy ebbs, as it must, to force physicians to stay calm. I turn heads as they continue to vomit. It will take hours of bathing, bottles of perfume, and even then, these odors will be sealed in my nasal hair. I sop purpling blood off shiny black leather mattresses. I core bulging blue veins with fourteen guage needles, massage fluid into them, postpone shock. Some nights I think I save a life. Larger, more physically agile trainees thump chests, it's before defibrillation is standard. Scurried, white-clad figures stuff sterile gauze into gasping abdominal holes. Sometimes a resident delicately slides writhing, sausage-intestines back in. I prefer the head, avoid lower body drama. I debride vomit, unstuff the mouth, learn to intubate. We, the subintern crew, slither impoverished patients down dark hallways, gaining momentum and experience.

I hear him moan, "She betta not be around when I get back." I push the tube down; then it's just his rasping efforts for breath. The weekend passion plays reverberate in me for years, follow me across the continent.

Tonight I lie in a white walled labor room in Colorado, gasping Denver's thin air between pains, as needy for oxygen as he was.

My belly bends me over again, centers me. I stretch around them, the sere contractions that shatter my will. I rock side-to-side in the bed. Motion relieves me some, like a hypnotic. I unclutch, uncurl, touch my abdomen, my fingers slope down its alien, hard surface. There were white tiled walls in the delivery suites in Philadelphia too, stained by uninterrupted screams. Women there delivered alone, without anesthesia, without a husband most nights, or family. Their anguish was more than physical, it harbored abandonment, injustice, and terror.

My first night on call in Obstetrics and Gynecology in Philadelphia, as a junior medical student, I attended an abortion. I hadn't time to think through ethics, political propriety, but I was certain, quietly certain, that a woman's body was hers. It was before moral points-of-view bannered above privacy. It was a simple, paternalistic society when I went to school, white bearded gods dominated every department.

Medical abortion was illegal.

I remember thinking stupid, unfair. I'd heard of wealthy women flying to Stockholm or Puerto Rico, to have safe, sanitary abortions. Two thousand dollars and up. My friends and I were not in that class. We attended college and medical school on scholarships, worked part time. I had two college classmates who survived coat-hanger jobs in our dorms. Lucky. Another had complications, a pelvic infection, raging fever, sterility. One hemorrhaged so badly she needed three transfusions.

It's three a.m., the room holds the chorus of *Eleanor Rigby*. It smells of alcohol and scrub-soap. We enter, gowned and righteous; I'm behind the resident. Our reddened hands drip, point up like prayers, away from our genitals. We are priest and priestess to the nurses in waiting, about to perform a mystic rite. They rush to assist us: towels, gloves, murmurs like gratitude or relief. As though they couldn't manage without us. We receive no reprimands for tardiness. The anesthesiologist is less forgiving. He cradles the woman's head on the table between his knees. The mother-almost-to-be.

Her eyes rove frantically, scan faces for comfort, a kind word, a clue. "Will it hurt?" She asks.

The resident snickers.

She darts her hand out and, with the accuracy of a snake's strike, clasps my clean, rinsed fingers in her hot, slithery ones.

"Now you're contaminated. You can't assist," a nurse hisses in my ear as she passes.

Inappropriate conduct flushes me, and I melt onto a stainless steel stool, adjacent to the table's head. Her hand's still got me, hot and tight. A mask slams over her lips. She gobbles sleep, her hand relaxes as the resident spreads her legs.

"All the lonely people," wails from the radio.

A smell like rancid fish oil pours from the vee of her split lower body. The residue of a botched attempt: forest green, thick yellow debris, with a crust of gray oozes; the air almost clots. A gelatin black blood clot accompanies a fractured miniature foot into the bucket below her pelvis.

Even the resident pauses, adjusts his grip on his stainless steel instrument, plunges his right hand with its metal extension back into her. While he's there, he sings, in synch, "leaving her face in a jar by the door, what is it for?"

Portions of lush red placenta, fragments of festering uterine lining follow into the steel pail. He scoops and sweeps, kneading her belly with his left hand, the other still buried deep inside. He reams and hums, a fingered limb is expelled, perfectly formed, black with gangrene.

"Aftercoming head," he says, stage whisper.

This is an obstetric description for breech deliveries, when the baby's largest, and last part, finally emerges. This man's making slide humor for himself. He has to reel his mind out of here, stabilize himself to continue. To save her life after an unsuccessful, home-style attempt, which got infected. One or two of these cases a week came to every ER in inner city hospitals across the country in the '50s and '60s. The combination of fetid odors, pieces of gore, and her fever glue me to the stool. I'm afraid to stand, afraid I'll fall.

A collapsed oval globe follows his outburst. There are black, unlidded eyes, glistening, wet hair, and two perfect pink ears.

I control myself, almost, grow still as the stool, rock very slightly with each fresh retrieval.

"A few more hours and she wouldn't have made it. It's marginal even now, so much sepsis," the resident shakes his head. "It's a crime."

I look down as my own abdomen rounds in a long, strong contraction. My baby swims between muscular convulsions. I am still conflicted, but not about having this child. I am loved. And married. I live divisive roles: wife/doctor. And now added responsibilities, mother. Will this overstretch me? A tripod positioning in different directions, I may permanently unbalance. Even my husband, who works in the laboratory with rat experiments, black and white facts, bar-graphs, scientific papers, is unable to reshape the grainy things that sprout between us; even he cannot re-ignite our early lust.

Pain yanks me back, centered in my pelvis. A giant, white coated obstetrician returns with an extremely long, stainless steel crochet hook. He uses it to rupture my steel-gauze membranes. Impenetrable to infection, or an emerging baby, they rip and flood the bed.

As if the metal invited a new level, a more intense, withering pain stabs. I swim sticky in the bed, fluid that cushioned my baby for nine months glues me to the sheets.

My husband and the doctor exchange three dirty jokes apiece, prepare to anesthetize me. I float back to girlhood, old wives at ancient kitchen tables, telling of women, aunts, distant cousins dying in childbirth. Covens whisper torture, undrugged deliveries, thirteen pound newborns. Nana taking my mother to a butcher shop for a scale large enough to weigh her, at one week of age. Greatgranny's loins so unhinged and swollen that walking was impossible for weeks.

My own mother's forty-eight hour active labor with me. I cringe in sudden guilt. She should have had a cesarean, but those were different times, the early forties. Women, ladies then, were not responsible. Only the father-to-be had the authority to sign for surgery on his wife. They owned their wives' bodies. My father was off in the Pacific fighting World War II.

It's the late '60s, things are progressive. Still, I'm more medicated, more sedated than I want. This twilight labor reminds me of the start, the startle recognition of too many missed periods. And the original doctor's barbaric pelvic exam. "You're too small. Your pelvis is android in shape; you won't deliver easily." Twelve hours and I haven't made sufficient progress. Maybe he was right. "Only a four pound premature will be deliverable without a Cesarean." My third delivery's a nine pound boy, who arrives rapidly, without assistance or complications, through my wrongly configured, too small space. Experts.

During this initiating labor, I'm still young, fairly obedient, and ignorant, despite my technical medical knowledge. I'm bedded in dependency and fear, both magnify my pain.

The huge round doctor enters again, wielding a needle. He inserts it deep in my spine. All "informed medical consent" in this era is filtered gibberish, medical pabulum. Lawsuits haven't yet begun in earnest. Truth is veiled. I am barely conversant with clinical medicine, graduated two months ago, so I let his hallowed hands rule me. They own and choreograph my first birth. I believe in their skill. A plastic tube is threaded into my spine; the juice runs in, my will runs out. I can no longer move my toes, knees, hips. The pain's replaced by numb paralysis. This is not an improvement.

I know from years of study, women no longer die in childbirth. That's true, isn't it? The doctor ungloves, ready to leave as I strike. My hand grabs for him, but I only get his coat hem. "Don't put me under a general, please. I'll be good, I won't scream, I promise."

The pain subsides and makes this statement more or less reliable.

"No matter what. Don't knock me out. Please."

He smiles knowingly. "Of course not, honey." Whatever I want to hear.

And what of his knowing? Second hand. Or third. Who would, could communicate this infantile terror, this cribbed prison of childbirth that bolts you on your back? His crafty hands strain at small heads, free gored placental pieces, repair maimed labia. These are not his native anatomy. The pain is noise in his ears. It does not penetrate his melody, that space of safety where his genitals reside, immune to birth-ripping.

The medicine succeeds where his words did not. I unknot, reel back to less conflicted, student days, when I was single. And one night in particular.

It was a navy November evening outside. I was in a gray, ill lit, labor room, at Temple Hospital, Philadelphia. I was the "doctor" then. More accurately, I masqueraded as one. I was only a junior medical student. This was my first exposure to Obstetrics. The nurses were busy, charting and chatting, so they sent me down to monitor a lady in isolation. Her room was at the far end of the corridor. An asthenic, languid woman bloated in the middle, writhed sinuously in a soggy bed. She was in advanced labor, with a murderously high temperature. I put cool, cinematically correct, compresses on her broiling forehead. I counted and recorded her rapid, thready pulse, made note of the slamming contractions as if I were back in physiology lab, recording the heart rate of the anesthetized dog. I unwrapped the wringing sheets, whispered calm, bland words. Inane. She watched me withdraw, heard me whistle a curtain between us. She rolled her head away, "A whistlin' woman and a crowin' hen, never do come to no good end."

I feigned professionalism, ignored her, hummed Nana's favorite, *Give me the moon over Brooklyn*, and buzzed for the nurse. She drowned my sound with a whistling scream.

"It's a comin'. Here it come."

I slammed the door open and called down the hall for help. I pulled her cage-bed with me, shoving long legs back into her own damp swamp. I thought if I managed her extremities, I could manage her whole-body behavior, even manipulate her experience of pain. Mind control was all the rage then.

I hoped I'd intuit what to do next. But life vulcanized her, and the heavy door slammed shut, shushed both of us.

I put the lights up, and she stopped struggling. Her screams subsided. All frantic activity was replaced by slow, heavy breathing, and childish whimpers.

I lifted the clammy, red streaked covers to a nauseous smell: feces, pus, and old blood. The odor pounded both of us. I wadded the sheet over the slop, and threw it on the floor, grasped the bed rail for stability, at the same time she did. She pulled herself up, glowered at me, eye to eye, whispered threats, obscenities, then promises in her fevered delirium.

I forced her down again, flat, my left hand on her forehead, my eyes scanned her body. Her belly wasn't as large. I twisted her hot, sticky thighs apart with my right arm. Her quads trembled with effort, trying to help, trying to hold her knees separate, to not mash my arm. Another whistle escaped, from me this time, as a small black mound pushed between her lips.

"Oh lord, here it comes," she screamed.

Now I was caged. I was the uneducated animal. My eyes scoured the room as if information might appear on the walls in code, or help leap from the slats of the venetian blinds. I jammed the buzzer with my hip and brought the baby's face up, off the bloody, soiled bed. Small shoulders slithered out, his bottom so slim it wriggled free, unassisted. He did not breathe. I had assumed that would be automatic, natural, somehow. But what was firm and pink seconds ago, a treasure, rapidly blued, grew limp and cold. I located his mouth despite a slippery white veil of vernix, removed a large red-yellow plug of mucous with my fingers; but still no breath.

I tilted him upside down, cradled his head in one hand, massaged his back and bottom with my other. His long white umbilical cord was still plugged into his mother. I crushed him against my chest for stability, his and mine. He began to warm. After what seemed like hours, he gasped and bellowed.

The mother was screaming again, lunged toward me. One endless leg dangled over the side of the bed. I smashed my thigh into it, pinned her solid. I showed her her son and she quieted.

I grabbed a compress near her head, that I'd used earlier to soothe her, and wrapped it around the baby's small shoulders. He pinked.

Pandemonium erupted through the door. Nurses, a resident, an intern, and two of my classmates arrived. Someone grabbed the infant, another, gowned, gloved, white coated, delivered the placenta. Someone else gave the mother injections, for sleep, for pain, and antibiotics.

The resident turned to me, smiled. "This wasn't a sterile delivery. You forgot to glove."

A refrain fluted over the room, "Where do they all come from? Where do they all belong?"

I touch her memory for luck. My labor's pristine in comparison. I have been religiously cleansed, had the enema, my pubis shaved of hair, no reminders that sex is associated with birth. These white walls are silent, except for Nana's song, *I'll be waltzing with Mazie / down Flatbush Avenue*. Time slips, thick ointment over a burn. By nightfall I'm less secure, the lonely-mother talisman, even Nana's protection, is less real.

It's eight p.m. before I dilate fully. I could be severed horizontally for all that I feel below my waist. One of those magic tricks run amuck, sawing through the coffin-box, the woman inside *is* cut in half. A rare spasm licks my bladder, still no back pain. I place my hands on my belly.

It's huge, hard as set cement. Without my fingers' touch, I no longer exist below my waist.

I was very alive there months ago. My husband and I were at a family celebration, escaped upstairs to a bedroom, away from the hospital and all that night-call, away from the party. We were greedy as we locked into each other, relieved momentarily of the solitude that siphons all lives. He whispered tender words, unconscious as I was of the new life we were whisking into the world. We stained the flowered bedspread, but I was unconcerned about mess then, just as it's irrelevant now. I embraced him with a kind of desperate hope, that we'd always love like this.

Then there were giddy, waiting months. Theoretically time to think and plan, but the demands of my senior year rolled anticipation and joy flat. I had the characteristic cravings, though. My diet swung wildly from normal: meat, salad, vegetables, fruit, to a package a day of double-fudge chocolate cookies, two black and white sodas, in addition to three balanced meals by the fourth month. Fifth month, I ballooned by forty pounds, spilled sugar in my urine. Gestational diabetes.

Bovine in sweet contentment and mastering lighter medical rotations, I swam through days and nights of sugar highs. I plummeted into frenetic, hypoglycemic shakes. Finally, I shivered to a physician, into management. He swatted me awake with a terrible literature of diabetic babies, complete with grotesque pictures. The statistics of abnormalities, stillbirth and retardation assaulted me. Guilt and terror replaced all craving immediately. I dieted, strictly. I was perpetually hungry. And tired. And scared.

Graduation terminated the lethargy of my senior year. It was sweltering that June. My parents and in-laws drove to Philadelphia for a dinner celebration, bickered over the seating arrangements at the restaurant. Their last levers of control dissolved in that heat. A new authority poked the front on my gabardine gown out, my husband and I, almost parents, were beginning to own ourselves.

That day falls away like gauze unwrapping as I'm rolled into the delivery room. I push and shove on command, spending myself with constipated exertion, to no avail. The spinal has unerringly paralyzed all nerves-to-muscles from what was my waist, down.

Gowned and gloved, my doctor husband and the obstetrician use huge, gleaming, semicircular blades, metal forceps, to clasp my baby's small, soft head, to pull her out. My pushes are useless. I hear, more than feel, the hollow, guttural suck as she's extracted, separated from me. My belly collapses, folds in on itself, like anti-matter.

This process is one end of a long, helical curl of separations that repeat for years, in less physical form. When I leave my daughter to return to work, the pain is not offset with an anesthetic in my spine. It's no more tolerable at fledging, when the children move to college dorms, and friends scold me that I have a career, shouldn't miss them so much. All these events are remote this evening.

Tori is whole. Five delicate fingers on each hand. I carefully, expertly examine her palms for signs of linear disarray that might spell mental retardation. There are none. I inhale deeply, study her face. Its curve sunshines the room, even though it is night. I rest on a pillow, my daughter sucks hard on my left nipple.

In the distance, the doctor remarks, "This will require at least fifty stitches."

Sutures I never even feel.

Everyone has discrete fields of interest in pediatric pathology, subunits of expertise. It's a closed clan of practitioners, and some pathologists gain authority studying a particular tumor; others research intrauterine infection, or developmental anomalies. In my case, the appeal was genetics. I have a natural affinity for peculiar details. Even minor anomalies that don't register with other docs are easy for me. Syndactyly, webbed fingers or toes, short, broad thumbs, the way a pinkie finger curls in, are things I always notice. Minute changes in hand features are often associated with serious internal disturbances. The axial triradius, the intersection at the wrist crease of overlapping palm circles, barely visible lines, can indicate a great deal about brain development. Today's medicine is dominated by sophisticated, technical studies, but still, I can read dermatoglyphics on a newborn's hand, confirm a syndrome, accurately, long before the chromosome results come back from the lab.

Naming

Names are like islands, which can change in meaning and time, both informing and absorbing environment. They have long affinity, like stepping stones, to the continent of the body.

When I was young, steepled in Catholicism, I chose *Faith* as my confirmation name, underscoring a pre-adolescent fervor. I'd gone to mass every Sunday from my first holy communion on, except summers; polio season. Some Augusts, the epidemics were so thick that people didn't let their child out in public.

Also, I fainted during Mass. The heat made this predictable, but I thought of it like a calling, dainty, romantic, a swooning for God.

Even then I wasn't a quitter. Someone would snap an ammonia capsule under my nose, and the acrid essence would reach me in that pink celestial space, serene and safe, no one hollering or hitting the back of my hand with a ruler, no one using a belt on my bottom, no one forcing me to kneel. The sunrays created a road from turquoise cumulus to the ground, God's highway, which vanished in that stringent stench. My mother's face, large and red above me because I had gotten special attention, would call my other name, and as soon as my knees locked, we returned to mass, took holy communion.

Faith was the first of the other trinity, the virtues, and I was full of them then, although I didn't know it. I believed I was sinning when I got angry with my parents, or was mean to my best friend, Irene Kopachinski. She and I walked to church after school every day that whole pre-confirmation year, a mile and a half each way through woods with muskrat and bluejays, robins and teens smoking. The trees in northern Jersey went bare by November, limbs iced and clicking through the winter. By spring, the marsh flushed wild with dark purple iris, tadpoles, and by late April, Baltimore orioles built pendulous nests in the quiet nile-leafed branches. I said the stations of the cross every day. So did Irene. She was adored by the nuns, smart and pretty, with long, swishy golden hair like the statues of Mary that weren't covered in veils. Mine was dark, I was gangly-limbed and wore oversized shirts to cover my body. Mother insisted I have home permanents every month, so my hair was tight to my head, fried. I didn't have a clue about sin or sex then. Not serious sin, or real sex. Anyway, I was going to become a nun when I grew up.

I recited catechism three days a week for the nuns, went to confession every Saturday, told *venial* sins first, then the mortal ones, like dipping a toe in a fast river, test the temperature, the priest's mood, *Bless me Father*. How much dare I say before he slams the grill shut and refuses me absolution. He could leave the confessional, drag me from behind the curtain, throw me out of the church forever. Flames licked my skinny shins, hot fingerlets melted flesh and bone. Eternal damnation.

How many sins can one small girl commit in seven days? I cursed a lot then, so I had plenty of kneeling time inside the confessional. I always got lots of Hail Marys for penance. I disobeyed my parents, I remember that, a constant, if not in action, in thought. I remember counting how many times on my fingers while I waited my turn in the pew. Only now, I can't recall why I disobeyed them. I remember how my mother loved Father Dougherty and would go only to him for confession; how one day, near Easter, I had new Mary Janes but couldn't wear them yet, she drove to church and talked to another woman in the parking lot. All the color drained from her cheeks. Her blue eyes blurred with tears, and her voice strangled. Father Dougherty had been sent away.

"Get back in the car. We're not going to confession today."

I started to argue, "What about holy communion? I can't take communion tomorrow if I don't go to confession. If I die I'll go to hell."

"Don't use that kind of language with me, young lady. And don't disobey. Get in the car; be quiet. One week won't kill you."

I did think mean thoughts about classmates too, and sometimes about my sister. Thinking in general was problematic in the church. Well, not just in the church for me, although I see now that they had that *where your thoughts go* right. *The body follows*, Sister chanted every Wednesday, the day she dealt with lust.

Curiosity, a virtue in science, where I later lost myself, is not applauded by organized religion, not Christian or Jewish or Muslim, anyway. Buddhism's different. But then Buddhism doesn't have GOD.

My thinking switched toward freedom in high school. I became friends, conversation-friends, with a boy a few years older, who was a Marxist. This was the '50s; people were still Marxists. My parents were Eisenhower Republicans, but Phil made me question everything, obedience, blind faith, God. I was hungry for ideas but flipped between extremes, saying rosaries, going to confession and communion, praying for guidance, and the recurrent seduction of questions. There was also my secret truth about my faith: a deep, deep doubt. Soon, even saying the rosary, like saying I love you, became disingenuous, its own kind of sin.

Those days of non-ecumenical Catholicism had lots of rules. A good Catholic could not attend another religious service; that sin hovered between venial and mortal, ill-defined, like Limbo. In my family this was a problem. My father was a Jew. We went to high holy days and Pesach at my grandparent's home. Orthodox. My sister and I went to Temple there too, the women and children hushed and segregated upstairs. It was always a kind of ecstasy to visit our cousins. Plus, our dad had asthma, but Uncle Al, his brother, did not. Al always tossed us high in the air, tickled me until I almost fainted from laughter, a playfulness and joy that didn't visit my parent's proper, clean house.

Once we got home again though, my sister and I had to go to confession, be cleansed from Pesach, or the synagogue. We had to make promises we weren't going to keep, to never attend a non-Catholic service again. Grandfather's Pesach's were close to high mass in terms of length, ceremony, and mumbled language. His Hebrew recitations began at sundown, chanted on until nine or ten, when matzo ball soup was served. Grandma fed all the children egg-noodles with butter and salt, and a wedge of raw onion in the kitchen first. We were better behaved after being fed; cousins who spent too little time together, our connections were precious.

There were visits during high school when I hoped my cousin and I had been switched at birth; I'd read of mistakes like this in the newspapers. Now that I was growing large breasts like her mother, it could be proved, and righted. Aunt Ruth was always smiling, alive and enthusiastic, and when she entered a room it smelled like lilacs caught in rain.

My grandmother herself smelled of east-European shtetl, and scalp. She was different from Nana in everything. Grandmother's hair was so long she only washed it once a month, wore it in a tight bun at her neck, but the free braid reached her knees. She kept it like that until she went into the home at ninety-five, and they cut it. Her hair, like my father's, stayed dark, with small streaks of white into her late eighties. Nana had short blue curls, tightly permed, and she splashed Chantilly perfume in her bosom, every day.

Grandmother wore an apron, even in the living room, smelling of onions and garlic and apricots, threadbare, and so soft you could lay your cheek against it and know her. She had bony hands with strong blunt fingers, and a gray-blue star-sapphire on her ring finger, above her wedding band. The stone bowed out like a belly, and in certain slant-light, its deep center was visible, radiating white lines like a blinking cross with stretch marks. It was set in yellow gold, with tiny diamonds, and I hoped when I married, I'd get something that exotic to study, in case I got bored. But it's a sin to lust after anyone's property. Plus, marriage would mean changing my name.

Ten Hail Marys

I should've considered Charity as a confirmation name. At eleven, I thought the word meant profligate giving, especially to the poor, easy giving, nudging toward too easy. Later, I went to the dictionary, learned it meant love. I was almost grown when I first fell, senior year of high school, hard and fast and true. Come fall, we went to separate colleges in different states. We wrote long lush letters; it was close to the end of innocence. We saw each other constantly over Thanksgiving break. John wanted to elope. I wanted to at least finish the semester. I was on full scholarship, enjoyed studying, loved learning. Besides, we were Catholic, reliable birth control was a distant landscape, forbidden to us by the church. We were wild in love, almost dumb in each other's presence, pawing, touching, testing, slurping mouths. He left by train before me, and I cried at the station, held Christmas in my heart.

Two weeks later he sent me a *Dear John*; he'd decided to become a priest. That lasted less than two semesters, but I never heard from him again; didn't learn about his marriage and begetting, for years. I never tried to contact him. Pride, one of the seven deadlies.

I got bursitis after the letter, so thoroughly my shoulder froze, and I needed a cortisone injection. I fainted as the liquid from the needle pushed the pain deep. I wore my arm in a sling all December; it was my right shoulder, a free pass from finals. I studied furiously after the holidays, bleak and full of self-pity. My scholarly fanaticism shocked my roommate, engaged at Christmas, her name about to change.

Make an Act of Contrition

After love tanks, work, travel, exercise or new love heals. But I didn't know remedies then, nor did I believe anyone else had ever loved like this. Years later, when my first marriage dissolved in a midnight rain, I stood threadbare and terrified to raise our three small children alone, forever.

My husband had hollered, *You don't respect me,* as he backed down the driveway. Then he rolled the car window up, went to her. Maybe he mumbled that, and I'd only imagined our shouts continued out of the house. His words stung, lack of respect was my line. He used the same accusation at Chanukah, when we "went out" to see if the thing was resurrectable. I was early thirties-horny; he was major-depression sad. Months later, divorced, we dated again. I needed two explanations now: why he'd never helped with the children unless friends were visiting, locking himself and his guitar in a room all evening as I cooked and bathed and played with them. Didn't he enjoy us? And why he'd decided, after ten years, to confess his string of infidelities. Did listing other names rekindle desire so he could make love to me, was I that bad?

Maybe my questions were too aggressive, but I was grasping for a connection, hoping we could save something, even something lame and tepid, like friendship.

His response was the first honest thing he'd said in five years. *I don't know why.* And that was true, like our love had been, singing and radiant at the beginning, when we were too young and overwhelmed to name it, too scared in our twenties to say the first I love you. *I really don't know why I left,* he said. *I just had to.*

Had I known how many times I would love, how elegant and ecstatic each fall would be, how addictive, I might have chosen *Charity*. If I'd known how crippling each demolition could become, I'd have been cautious, maybe I would've considered *Chastity*. Ignorance has its own edge though, and benefits.

At eleven I was slapped across the cheek by the bishop, *Faith*. I see its importance now in retrospect, in my whole life, how closely aligned it is to hope, really, and how both are blind. I see it especially in the context of work.

There's a religious comfort in a consuming career, particularly if you can kid yourself you're doing good, performing a mitzvah with your effort. And if your work involves children, the seduction's slicker. I was a pediatric pathologist for thirty-five years. A lot of devotion and dedication to correct diagnoses, to try and save children's lives, and a lot of autopsies to delineate diseases and malformations, assign specific highly accurate names, and to give answers to families. A lot of karma. A lot of discipline.

During those years of medical training and practice, I married twice and shared their names. Both husbands were smart and sexy and drop-over handsome. They carved pleasure and passion in me; even in that pre-soulmate era, we were connected. Molecules of each mainman embedded in me, splinters, but not the festering kind. I know the body walls off foreign, circles the strange with inflammatory cells, fibrosis, giant cells. I've studied the slides all my life. I like to think of their residues as incorporated, almost-accepted self.

My first husband's family was Jewish; not very, I later discovered, but when I came in, there was pressure for me to convert. His mother's family had kept Kosher in her youth, even though her father ran the meat concession at Macy's and could have gotten cheap, wholesome food, wholesale. That family had three strapping boys, big eaters. It took an arrest of the local Kosher butcher, for selling traif meat before the old ways loosened. Still, a Shiksa, even one with a Jewish dad, was none too welcome.

His father seemed more open, but that was surface. He was a blood-researcher in medicine, and had been a wild-eyed progressive in youth, a registered Socialist in the twenties, investigated by McCarthy in the '50s. He was Jewish, but Reform.

I took serious Judaism conversion classes two evenings a week, the entire second semester freshman year, when I should've studied biochemistry and physiology. When we visited my fiancé's family, their entire culture was new to me. They had a maid who served dinner; everyone regaled one another and dined, instead of sitting on a plastic-wrapped couch in front of TV trays, staring flicker-faced at the new American altar. I was eager to embrace my husband's name, with its medical pedigree, his Dad, a three-time nominee for the Nobel. Also, I had "issues" with my own father, so I happily shed his last name. I was proud to become a goodwife. It was 1965.

The converting Rabbi was dictatorial; I would take the name Ruth, whither-thou-goest-Ruth, as my conversion name. In no time I was reinvented, like a state witness.

During the conversion ceremony itself, I remembered studying with a priest, senior year of college, to try and reconnect with Catholicism. My struggles over faith then involved conversations which reminded me of how Mother always spoke of Father Dougherty's kindness. This priest had that same kind of patience. We dissected Catholic doctrine he'd made me read, but still, my mind could not split God. One, or a million.

Late May he said, "If you're born Catholic and lose your faith, you're condemned to hell for eternity. But if you're born Buddhist or Protestant say, and convert to Catholicism, then change your mind, and follow the precepts of whatever you convert to next, you just have to do a little penance in Limbo. Then you can go to heaven." It sounded something like explaining original sin, which could be wiped away like a baby's vernix caseosa, cleansed early, with Baptismal oil and prayers. "I'm not sure about all that," he continued. "I mean it is canon, but still. You're a spiritual person, very spiritual, but you're not Catholic. If you could accept the trinity, and just have trouble with the virgin birth say, we could still give you sacraments, communion, last rites. But you must accept Jesus and the Holy Ghost, and of course, the Father, as one and only one God." He offered to speak to my parents, he meant Mother, but I knew there'd be hell to pay and I said I should tell them. He then asked if I wanted a writ of excommunication.

Try to eat meat on Friday: gag

Mother's reaction was more violent than Dad's outbursts, which had peppered my childhood, and my sister's. Mother, always afraid of what the neighbors knew or saw or heard, ran screaming out of the house on a blue spring day, banging the screen door wide, swinging her arms as if swatting huge insects or bats, her housedress flapping around her shins. "If only you'd become a whore. I could understand that, I've always expected it." I stood still, very still, grabbed the edge of the doorsill, hoping the closing screen would smash my fingers, deform them. I was a virgin, trying to tell my truth, like Nana had instilled in me in Brooklyn. *Just tell what really happened, honey. No one will ever get mad at you if you're honest.*

Later that evening, after I'd made and cleaned up supper, my father's gray face hard marble, his asthma inhaler in use all afternoon, after he'd calmed her enough to get her back inside the house, Mother wept, "Oh Milton, do you think we should take you to the hospital?" Her voice was ruined, her beautiful skin, tear-streaked. Neither of them said a word to me.

Just before bed, he slammed my door open. "You've broken your mother's heart. She believes she'll be eternally damned for this."

"But it's my decision. In fact, it's less a decision than a confession. I can't believe in the three-in-one God thing. If any soul will be punished, it'll be mine." He shut the door so carefully I never heard the latch. An old pattern.

It was a one day event. No one ever broached the subject again.

My second husband, Lamar, was Mormon. No improvement. I was considerably older when I married him, if not chronologically, then by experience. I'd finished my training, passed boards, had had a tubal ligation, owned my own home and car, had three very young, suddenly insecure children. He didn't demand conversion about God, but eventually, about near everything else. By the time we married, my medical career was established; a name change, professionally, was out of the question. Socially, I thought the entire rigmarole silly, but he didn't. I don't honestly know if it was a possession thing, his paternalistic heritage, or willful, but he pushed and pushed and after the *Achile Lauro*, when an old Jew in a wheelchair was summarily dumped into the sea because of his passport name, I agreed.

I'd changed my last name twice after the first divorce, long before I remarried. Once, as a sort of feminist fashion-statement in the mid-'70s, I hyphenated it, confused everyone. I'd go to the dry cleaners, or register at a hotel, and I'd either be listed as an R or a W. It was roulette; hardly the sophisticated move I'd imagined. My children's friends always called me Mrs. R, immutable, even today. For simplicity's sake, I eventually deleted my first ex's last name, switched back to my root.

But here's the thing about changing names: you get lost. I mean, by thirty or thirty-eight, you know who you are surely, but then, late one dozy afternoon, at an international conference in pediatric pathology, I'm at a cancer session and an intriguing paper presents five cases of adrenocortical carcinoma in children. It's a very rare tumor. The young man references an article from a pediatric journal I subscribe to. His discussion sounds familiar. He sites an earlier report of two cases of this cancer, with unique liver abnormalities. With growth disturbances. Associations of rare disorders, unusual couplings, are my passion. In medicine. *No such thing as coincidence,* my mentor taught me early, then hired a statistician to teach reason, probabilities, and question that first rule. Original beliefs though, especially if they appeal to temperament, are hard to eradicate. The presenter mentioned the authors of the original paper, someone et al. I've read the article, the details ring bells.

After he's applauded, I approach the lectern, ask for the reference. Rosen et al. I was that Rosen.

Give your silver rosary to Nana

I often think of both my grandmothers as they aged. Two women from different religions, strong and willful in youth, sworn enemies for decades. I watched their family-war, installments of our own soap opera, until they hit their late seventies. Then, the old women, the only ones left, leaned toward one another on summertime porches, almost deaf, toothless and cranky, talking each other home.

Their gnarled hands rested in their laps; neither raised a fist any longer. Grandma, Father's mother, had knitted for her grandchildren as soon as her first was born: two sweaters for my cousin, one for me. Mother's mother,

Nana, crocheted until her vision failed. If it was a sing-a-long-evening, they'd rock on the porch, their voices high and crackled, like taffeta rubbing itself. Those were nights Nana spun her thumbs around each other, whirring time. They'd seen so much, those two, flappers in youth, bound-breasts hard against ribcages because the fashion was to look like boys. They recalled the first time they saw a horseless carriage; which apartment had the first radio in their tenements; how they'd seen a man walk the moon. And they were friends now, because they were the only ones who understood.

Even in high school, dreaming life, stalking love, I used to pause near each of them when we visited, trying to imbibe who they were. In age, all their vitriol is folded away. Not senility, not at all, just conversation and a kind of closeness, a soft-edged clasping, like fingering an old postcard, the address barely legible, ink smudged from too much touching. You can't read the signature, but there, in the lower right hand corner's the name. And just above it, in blue ink: *Love*.

My baptismal name's Patricia, Ireland's patron
saint, rumored to have run all snakes into the sea

Love-need is something I may never outgrow. I still want it, especially at holidays, or family gatherings, when everyone is coupled. No matter how egregiously.

Maybe it's habit. I was wed through most of my twenties, thirties, and forties. Different men, different names, but married. And while I know in my secret heart that I have never been as consistently happy or stable as I am, living alone, I still yearn for coupling. It's not the companionship my women-friends pine for. And I don't at all mind going to a restaurant alone. I hate talk during a movie, so I don't need a companion then either. But sex, ah sex, I miss. And it's more than that. It's wanting to be special to someone; wanting to be wanted, and important, and cherished. It's loved I want to be. Charity, not pity.

The second marriage soured. One day Lamar simply stopped listening. June 20th, 1989. He heard what I said, could've spouted my words back, but he was no longer affected. Just like that.

I tried hard to win him back, at least his attention, but when love leaves, your mind and body, your personality, evacuates. You yourself become emotionless as a cheese-grater, hard and sharp with a thousand surface holes, before you fracture. And after, there are bits of you strewn over the years, bloodied, confounded, gauzed as a bandaged archipelago.

After Lamar's withdrawal, I got sick. First, rheumatoid arthritis. I worked for a boss who was as secretive as my husband then. Both men described themselves as shy, but they were hidden, a little devious. Also they shared an identical shade of shale-blue eyes. I got confused. Or maybe it was the way color drained from those eyes to sink-gray, when they dissembled. Working with arthritis was grueling, almost impossible. My feet swelled first and I could barely balance. I no longer took the stairs down three flights to the OR to confer with the surgeon. I had to ride the elevator up to the lab to freeze specimens. I either sent a resident down with the report or called the OR myself, not as satisfactory as examining the surgical field first-hand, talking face-to-face with the surgeon. Plus, this slowness added anesthesia time for the child. I bought thick soled shoes then, a size larger than normal, and my knees bulbed like spring plants in sunshine.

Then my hands, ohmygod, my hands. They weakened until I could no longer manage the Stryker saw, couldn't use bone scissors, and finally dexterity went. I'd always prided myself that thoracic surgeons, neurosurgeons even, came to the morgue periodically to watch me dissect. And I didn't know if it was from all those years of numbing routine, or the swelling and deformities that accompanied arthritis, or from a kind of soul-soreness, but teasing tissue under a dissecting microscope, handling miniature scissors and forceps, was no longer possible. It was as if I'd grown paws.

One day my hands were so red and swollen I couldn't sign the surgical reports without wincing. "I'm taking sick leave," I said to my partner, "to see if the arthritis will calm down."

Everyone had suggestions then to treat the disease: no sugar, cut out caffeine, no nightshades, acupuncture. Stop eating wheat. Don't add salt. It's alcohol; it's your attitude; it's stress. But when I said I was leaving medicine, my partner said, "Maybe it's the wrong place to leave, maybe you should leave home." He stood in my doorway, watched my whooping crane mobile circle my head, rubbed his beard. "Maybe you're quitting the wrong thing." He knew me. We'd worked together long, long days for twelve years. Our offices shared a very thin wall.

I took six months off, took heavy drugs, gold, Plaquenil, prednisone. Lamar and I moved to his Aspen condo to renew our relationship. I had acupuncture every week, took daily long naps, did visualizations, smudged the condo, but nothing worked.

I lost weight then, so much I needed two towels under my bum to sit in a bath. Size two was perfect in my husband's mind, and my sister and women friends were green. I'd never really had weight problems, but this was ridiculous. Finally, I was diagnosed with cancer.

That was one nutty summer, 1991. I had biopsies and staging and finally a radical hysterectomy. I separated from my husband then, found a cancer support group. Over half those women separated from their man, regardless of their prognosis. Not what I thought people in relationship with critical diagnoses would do.

One day, after I was a little stronger, still recovering, I bragged to my sister I'd started to gain weight again. She said, "God's gonna punish you for that." I pointed out he probably already had.

After my six month cancer-free follow-up, I finally, finally left Lamar. I'd separated from him several times, come back; left, reunited. Lamar was a fighter pilot, a warrior, and I was weak with arthritis and then cancer. He was deeply humiliated in front of his friends that I would leave. He sent two dozen roses a day and chocolates, dark chocolates, which my sister and daughters insisted I refuse. In private, when we got together, it started out sweet, he was initially solicitous, but then grew vindictive, hollered, shook me, threw things. He had perfect aim. I was still a doctor at heart, full of my own kind of hubris. I honestly believed I could control him.

On the seventh leave, as if I'd memorized a manual for abused wives, I stayed gone. But I loved him, hard and long and hoped for years, even after that divorce, that he'd change. In a way, not so different from my mother's responsibility for my soul. If I'd modeled love better, a gentle, patient love, instead of the passion we shared, he might have "caught" my behavior-paradigm like an infectious disease, chicken pox, or measles.

I still feel raw without him. It's been a dozen years. I miss his arms, a bandaged protection that, when removed, exposed fragile, nude skin and alien geography.

Hope. I think that's the last virtue to go. It's a hard one. You can relinquish faith, just open your palm and let the belief that you'd questioned anyway, float.

You can close up shop on love too; age reduces hormones, and all that jealous craziness. There are hurts that don't heal fully, but time fades the intensity, at least. And desire drowns in the everyday; we all learn that. But hope, that's another thing entirely. Without that, what's the difference between warm flesh and a cadaver?

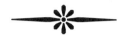

For years I worked every third Saturday, processing surgicals, reviewing the hardest cases of the week, doing autopsies, teaching residents and fellows. One beautiful sunny April Saturday, the resident called me from my office to plan the photographic documentation of five specimens. There were four tiny skin-cups of fingertips. Black. The identifying whorls and arches, perfect dermatoglyphics, stood in high relief on each tip. There was also a complete distal index finger, nail included. Badly charred, surgically severed. The three year old had explored the smooth, slick surface of the new ceramic stovetop, accidentally left on.

ER Euphemism

Be brave, I say, don't move, I'm sorry to hurt you.

She's limp, tiny, too quiet. The ER's a flame of activity and there's no nurse's note. The young mother weeps, the knot of her curls over her child in the curtained space.

I cup my hand under the child's head, the size of a small cantaloupe, the same woody skin with pliable, doughy interior. It's hard to remove the tangle of her from her mother's limbs.

It's dark, Mommy. Mommy, where are you?

Touch the occipital curve and the child's face becomes a wrinkled map: pain, fear, compliance. There's a family resemblance, the lift of the eyes, the set of the mouths, only the child is so much thinner her cheeks mold in.

The child asks again for light.

The nurse appears now, sterile gauze to the wound under pressure, something congeals on the scalp. Something knots behind my eyes. *Suspect NAT*, the nurse whispers, our small, medi-speak conspiracy, *Non-Accidental Trauma.*

I strap the child to the gurney, swab her elbow hollow, fresh alcohol careens through Saturday night's arena. The IV runs in, a lullaby leaks from my lips, I lean low, beside her ear and tell her.

What, what can I possibly say.

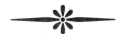

Senior year of medical school I worked the wards and ER at St. Christopher's Hospital for children in Philadelphia. One Saturday night a five year old presented with a huge, stinking, black bandage on her hand. The mother was very loud, very, very angry. "I told her to stop sucking her thumb," she said. "She's defiant." I unwrapped the bandage. There was a gangrenous thumb, jet black, with green pus, below the filth. The child never shed a tear.

Madness: A Vivid Interior Void

Payne Whitney, New York City, 1972
The first week is white. Thick in isolation. Absence of connection with anyone, anything, even color, makes it elongate. It stretches, a parabolic curve, around my breathing that continues, willed or not.

The white spreads like excrement from a skywriter, belching cloud clots, burying the sky.

The first smell is sex. Aging stale mushrooms, musty fish. It creeps up from under rigid bed linens, vice tight. Rough muslin like hospital issue anywhere, only more constrictive. The orderlies here have forced fragments of steel wool into these sheets. I know because any skin that surfaces gets abraded. Red sores pus over and this perfume mingles with the sex scent. The sheets chafe even my private, pinioned parts. Movement is remote as thought. They have clamped heavy canvas straps over the linear strings of chenille bedding. They subdue me further with injected drugs. So often that I miss the light/dark shifts that must occur behind chalk-white shades.

When I do move, it's a moan. Captive, defeated, unable to believe my senses. The first birth is loss. My son, tow-headed toddler, explodes through my head with laughter and need. He's hurtled to an earlier day, his rose mouth leeched tight at my nipple. He sucks nurture from me, nervously, fast. Time slips through my skin like translucent blue-white silk, my own milk runs down the side of my breast. I will not feed him again.

The days of the week thin. The smell is cow milk now, curdling in my hair, sweat-stuck to the pillow. When my eyelids finally scrape back, I no longer see road-map veins, just the coffin of satin light from the window: long and narrow. It mirrors the shape of my white iron bed, edges sharp and angled, reinforcing regularity, in this wired, paned, untouchable world. The rectangular room reflects this too, all walls drenched in snow.

Mornings, the plaster ripples. Late afternoons the sun enters, heats things up, the walls pulse, move closer and closer, almost clap. Another attempt to obliterate me.

The high ceiling contains an eye. A central, weak bulb observes me from its circled, cream colored casing. It blinks on and off, as my days must. It records my cycles, my drool. Late at night, without these distractions, I wonder if I eat or sleep, shit or pee. Surely there would be other colors, different odors, if...

It must be Tuesday when I recognize the light as a window. I start to study it. I am still flat in bed, stitched in the shroud of sheets. The sill paint peels in crusts of gray white. The grime on the pane protects my retina from the blinding August sun that bleeds in late morning, even in this city. I try to observe carefully enough to determine if the dirt is inside or out, dust or rain. The drugs make focus on this kind of minutia, whether through the eye or mind, impossible. They stun movement, shatter thinking with the indiscreet corrosion of a vat of sulfuric acid tossed at random.

My vision's irreversibly blurred, my speech dissociated and incoherent. When I will my body to move, it lurches, so my shadow's a stilted silhouette caught in strobes. My tongue cleaves to the roof of my mouth, my legs freeze in preparation for a single step. My arms stop midair, refusing to syncopate like normal appendages. My body's stiffness precludes even the idea of an embrace. It also prevents the most primitive self-protective reflex, a hand raised before a face to ward off a slap or a punch.

Equally profound, but more subtly destructive, is the chemical weight of phenothiazides on thought. Try to integrate information, recall a specific detail, try to reason, observe for more than a nano-second, impossible.

I snap focus: black vertical bars on the window spear me. Long ago there were stripes, horizontal venetian blinds then, on the windows of Nana's home. Other lines, a pale blue-striped pinafore, made by her hands. I stand in her shadow in that hanky light dress, smocked by her fingers. She knew the magic of a needle and thread, pinched material in symmetric puckers like an old lady's face, the way it creases toward the mouth, parched lips waiting a lifetime for one particular kiss.

The lines of that cotton pinafore reside in me somewhere, but current lines repeal youth, summertime, possibility. The small top lay soft on my nipples, stitches pricking ever so lightly. The billowed skirt swung free from my no-hips. Naked long legs ran, skated the wind. Cropped summer heat, harvest-ready barley, ripe sunflowers, grazed me. I twirled giddy.

Another nurse enters me with her syringe. I never hear the numbing, medicine-rich, white-clad women enter. They float on shadowed feet. What were details of truth evaporate. The needles blur, sew old times to the forgetfulness of now. A glistening vacancy, achromia, recurs behind my lids, spreads over me, slows my mind. A question occurs, a thing I want to ask, need to know. Where am I?

Then I understand, even understand *why*. I'm scrubbed. I'm in an old fashioned surgical suite. The 19th century kind. A long oval amphitheater where decks of observers encircle the patient and doctors. Witnesses are separated by glass so blood and disease will not spatter them. Because of this boundary, any possible disruption, or disgust, on the part of onlookers will not distract the concentration of the surgeon-barbers. I hold my scoured hands up for the honey colored gloves to be snapped into place, my palms open to accept the scalpel of power.

But no, I am the patient. Strapped and stripped on the table, I'm already incised. The terror's so intense it obliterates pain. I shiver with cold and fear. If Nana were here she'd share her crocheted shawl, ease the ivory spiderweb design around my shoulders, shoo away the chill. The edges would close over my exposed body, brush my legs. The sweet residue of her vanilla flesh mingled in the fibers would staple courage into me.

I see myself reflected in the overhead surgical light, look hard for the microphone hidden in the rim. The steel border reflects my body in a curved manner, the distortion's like a bent mirror in a circus. There's a longitudinal, full body incision: an autopsy. It's my due. I'm a pediatric pathologist and now I'm going to know how it feels, this scientific duty I perform daily on infants, fetuses, children, adolescents; it's my turn.

I'm opened from my sternum, just below my neck, to my lower abdomen, right at the pubis. The slice is vertical, crisp, almost bloodless. At the bottom there's a mangle of dark maroon jelly congealing with kinky black hair. Many organs have already been removed, probably for donation. My liver, kidneys, intestines. The odor from that last hamburger mixes with the acid of digestion, I can almost taste the putrefaction. There's a pale slippery snake of bowel, milking food through, and oversized pink coffee beans, kidneys, processing the last sting of urine. My crimson liver manipulates a myriad of internal and external chemicals, detoxifying, reconstituting my essence. They all ooze scant clear serum and dots of blood in individual, sterile, stainless steel pans. I remain prone on the table.

There are the two salmon pillows, arching symmetrically like cathedral windows, in a separate container. They gasp air in, wheeze the smut of betrayal out, like old fashioned, hand-worked bellows. And there, in an adjacent tray, is my heart. Ruby muscle streaked by yellow fat, a thick walled machine, which still beats, pumps one last time to process all the emotional excesses: my life. It continues to perfuse oxygen to the brain, futile, an attempt to have me think clearly. It must be some primitive drive to hold life together a little longer, despite all these separated parts. It's too late, I know that. But my heart continues to beat, pure reflex, a galvanic response. I study it and recognize the ice-shock of the metal pan bypassing normal nodal circuitry. Irregular twitching occurs; it only resembles contractions.

I try to understand this. Get lost in the heart's control mechanism, electric circuitry, currents, too close to physics. Then I remember the forest of theft. I didn't authorize these removals; I never signed a release. There must be a mistake. If this is an autopsy, I'm dead. No one can survive without these organs. They're not extraneous like tonsils or an appendix, they comprise me. Yet I experience this. I'm still here. But not completely.

I watch all of this mesmerized, fascinated, terrified. I've always feared fanaticism. It figures true-believers would vivisect me. I observe each removal with split attention, a familiar posit. When things become intolerable, destroy who I am, I flee. I've always done this, divided into a peripheral witness and a semi-conscious participant. This time I watch from the top of the room margins and some part compiles a record. I turn to the audience, those piled in the bleachers behind the shield of protection, and scan spectators for signs of discomfort, compassion, betrayal. Both my parents are there, nodding subdued approval. My husband's slavering with erotic revenge. My boss paces the back row, wrings his hands, distraught. Nana's bereft, weeping, weary. It was her compliance with my husband that finished me. She listened to his reasons with her head.

My babies teeter on a low row, glued to the specter. Please don't let them see me disemboweled, splayed open, so empty. Please, take them away. Let them know I love them. Do what you must to me. Let them be.

Just as I cannot hear any commotion or distress because of the glass partition, they, happily, cannot smell my fear. Nor the putrid, sweet cadaver scent that I'm becoming. They cannot hear the chorus of cherubic voices encouraging me to relax, trust, to lie back and enjoy. Several ethereal commands dart in and out as my ears uncouple. Twin voices sing reassurances, insist this is for the best, it will turn out fine in the long run. That I will indeed be different, but better. Reconstructed. Their melodious sound belies the ominous tremor that begins to move my bones.

I'm on the cold steel table, thin rivulets of blood trickle down my sides; this convection further cools me. I vibrate centrally as the bone saw whines, and they open my spinal column. I smell the warm mix of disc dust and blood, a familiar odor, permanently imbedded in my nasal hair from the hundreds of autopsies I've performed. But this time it's distinct, it's me smelling me. It's less acrid, less burnt. More like thick maple syrup. Binding.

Suddenly, it's clear. I understand. I am to receive the first brain transplant. I am so fucked up this is the only solution. Relieved for a second because they will return all my other organs, I filter back to my eviscerated body. Another mistake.

The voices begin in earnest now. Some wail like hired Irish mourners, remind me this is a tragedy. But I don't feel sad. In fact, I feel nothing. I am paralyzed, ransacked, almost extinct. Someone whispers that he will forevermore direct me through my future, all I need do is let him lead. Follow his instructions. A screechy, high pitched voice insists I obey her regulations, learn her rules. Just like life. But for the now, all I have to do is lie back and not interfere. Spread my legs, did you say? Someone whispered that directly into my pelvis.

They've loosened my spinal cord, they're shaving my head. They remove my hair, that barricade of rebellion I flaunted through years of medical training. This tether linked me, for an extra few choruses, to my own song. My long hair swayed behind, hiding hips that rarely found time to grind.

After awhile, I barretted it into submission, hoping to earn respect in the rigid society of physicians, a bastion of male precision, perfection, propriety. A medical career purports a mix of art and science, to produce healers. Actually, medical training spits out shells, years of life buffed away in study. I knotted my hair on top of my head then, as though the added height would crown me equal to the men. Ninety-two percent of physicians and medical students were male in the '60s. Some days I wore a pony tail, others, a thick single braid. Controlled, untouchable, like rich dark fur swept into asexuality. I became the frozen bland woman, pince-stepping the wards of commandos. I sanitized my animal origins while my male colleagues spewed raw sexuality all around, bragged and strutted in front of nurses and female patients.

These same men are using the saw on me now. They cut a gently curving arc, enter my skull. I feel excruciating pressure, a heaving pull, which detaches the upper skull cap from the base. They're in my cranium, severing all neuronal connections. With a final lunge of will power, I eject to the ceiling.

But it's too late. I've been snagged. The rip of bone from bone reels me back. Now the cold slick edge of the scalpel rends all nerves running to my face. I will be expressionless. There's blind groping on the underside of my brain, gloved fingers move gyri and sulci, blunt dissect small nerves from cerebral insertions, snap the optic tract, clamp vessels. I feel nothing, see nothing, but still hear many things.

The first sounds are the scrape of chair legs outside my door. It's later in the bleached week. The tilted chair and his dark shades implode my crystal solitude. His smoke eases in, roams around my room. I hear the scratch of denim near his crotch as he approaches my bed. He rips through a plugged silence, removes bandages from my ears. I blink, but he's only readjusting his balance on his stool. A study in cool.

Then his hot cigarette breath's on my neck. I catch a bead of his sweat on my tongue. It just formed on his forehead, would have plunged between my breasts if I hadn't caught it. It tastes of virility. He leans over me again, rakes his hand through my hair, adjusts the pillow, slips the straps off for awhile, lets my body breathe. He slips under the white cotton blanket for a solitary contact, flicks my clit, then he's gone. Back at the door, stationed to prevent suicide. It was stabilizing somehow, his touch.

I begin moving. Diaphanous, I sail the long corridors, streaky as a cirrostratus cloud. I almost flow, slender curling lines, like freshly spilled milk. I cringe in corners at the smallest sound. I memorize the floor plan, slip along the ceiling where organic residue of rancid meals crust. Nothing's near as pure as the whitewash proclaims. I can smell the faint mouse odors of fucking in an occasional closet. I hear the static of all-night television, the blue gray haze it emits, further short circuiting our drug-destroyed minds.

I eavesdrop, catch wisps of nursing reports, hear furtive tattles of orderlies: room 103's aberrant tonight, 408's screaming obscenities again. An organized spiral of surveillance. I'm so swift and silent that I'm ignored. I watch the pervasive watching.

There's the deep, authoritative, male voices of the doctors, housed in a special room with huge block letters marked STIFF. No, maybe it says STAFF. Where the bloody hell did I leave my glasses? Only M.D.s are permitted to congregate here. The accumulated data on inmates is regurgitated to them, regularly. So they know. Or can. But in this clandestine room, their chatter revolves around nurse Mary's tits or Barbara's ability to give head. They barely expose their patient's charts, let alone delve into problems, some of which are so similar to their own, they're threatening beyond insoluble. Their glib attitudes almost shield them. They are ivory-towered, clearly superior, so they have the keys. And the drugs.

I slither inside their cave, after all I have an M.D., too. I shiver in the subzero temperature, a ghost at the edge. These managing men are unctuous, privileged, pompous. I post myself at a three planed intersection, the high left-hand corner of ceiling and walls. Secured by real boundaries, I don't need to flee further, although my recurrent temptation to run, ripples through me.

I scan the faces of men who control my fate. I used to belong to their fraternity. Well, sort of. I was only a girl. I used to wear a white coat. Now, I'm in a long-armed white jacket. The sleeves wrap around my middle, swaddle me. If they unloop them I could spread my arms, beat them furiously, fly.

If they unbound my belly, they would see the inept primitive sewing some hack surgeon did after he returned my abdominal organs. There are huge uncomfortable knots of thread connecting the center of me. I still have a gaping hole in the middle of my belly, an aureole of ache rings this. I try to move my arms, to circle my hands towards this gap, but nothing responds. It's then I remember they severed all my nerves.

I'm in the ceiling corner, still as marble, ashamed that I continue to eavesdrop on these spies. Finally, hours into the droned rounds, I will my body away. I feel pithed and flaccid, the way we ruined frogs, destroying spinal cords in biology 101.

I fly down a central corridor, see the inmates. Zombies shuffle with mannequin stolidity and blank faces, sit at tables covered with white linen cloths, eat gray food. They are drugged beyond repair, no longer whimper protests. I am one, or will be soon, if my restraints are eased. I'm back in bed, in my body, clasped into white again, under cover.

Later, new voices claw me.

"Get yourself some pride, girl. Get your lazy ass up. If you're going to be a whore, do something. You can't just lay there all day, get up, hear?"

"I can't. Nothing works. I can't even raise my middle finger." I slouch deeper into my body.

"It's okay, you're trying. We'll set you up with Al here. He'll watch out for you, get you clothes and dope. You just got to do like he says. Start by spreadin' your legs, honey."

I grunt against the stifling bedspread, the cloying voices, but all effort, even just paying attention, exhausts me. I'm gone, again. It's dusk when I get back. The room's dim, city lights blink through the window grease. Then I see it's not a room, it's a huge amphitheater.

I flee again, ricochet between the borders of the ceiling-wall and the flat body. I stop abruptly. The transplant's complete and it's a miracle: there's no rejection. I'm in recovery, in the white week. Weak, altered, placid. I don't know what's been returned, what's been rearranged, what remains vacant. Perhaps I never will.

But I have work again, can feel life through that. I will learn their rules, spin the sentences they want to hear. I will improve. Never mind it's their definition of sanity, their idea of getting better, they're the shrinks, construct normal, write the texts. I will earn a release, get back with my children again. It will take time, there will be voices, years of voices, there will be visions, constant struggle, but none as bizarre, clairvoyant and radically obliterating as this.

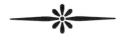

Courage is a heart-virtue, but I associate it with hands too. Two years after my break, I got very sick in the middle of the night, needed an emergency "session" with my psychiatrist. Michael, my first husband drove me, and I actually asked to be rehospitalized. It was a full moon; all the mental wards and hospitals in Denver were full. My shrink dosed me heavily on Stellazine. He cupped the vial over his desk after our session, and Michael reached forward, but my psychiatrist said, "No, it's her disease, her responsibility." My hands shook as he rolled the vial into them; enough pills to kill me, to stop respiration in a whole family.

Years later, my doctor told me he had had a patient suicide once, that he hadn't slept at all that night. It was his belief in me that changed things, though; I couldn't let someone down who trusted me that much. There was a bed the next morning I no longer needed.

LAPSE

I was forty before I began to appreciate Mozart or kindness. Neither interested me when I was first in your arms, Michael; pleasure held me tight. Your words kindled me until something shifted; we soured, the way an incompletely wrung dishrag does, day after day. Your voice tamped as you withdrew into silences long and stingy, a drumming.

Tonight I'm at a condo party in Cherry Creek; it's the late-'90s. I eavesdrop on a war weary marriage, a Sicilian couple, my neighbors, display their tactics for the crowd. He's drunk and quarrelsome; she's a head taller, has perfect posture and a serene face like ivory porcelain. He hollers at me across the table, over the hum of conversation. His wife moves next to him, as if proximity provides purchase, or safety. Her eyes are kohl-lined, a little blood-shot. I hear him, although I'm chewing ice cubes, that sound loud and close and grinding. There's a cold, sharp pain in a back molar.

"So doc," he shouts, "Do you write prescriptions?"

"No, I don't do that–"

"Well, but you are a doctor, aren't you?"

The room quiets. She chain-smokes unfiltered Camels. He lights her next cigarette without even looking. She inhales slowly, then glides away.

"But I'm just a pathologist," I say. I always sound apologetic about this. In medicine, I'm an encyclopedia of information, respected. Outside the hospital, my study of children's diseases and deaths makes me a different kind of human. Small ghost corpses surround me, insulate me from normal. Even you were suspicious. I sip my Perrier with its twist of lime, cover the sore tooth with my tongue.

He calls back again, "So doc, I went to the doctor today and you know what he said?"

Oh, I'm not up for this. I should respond with *No, I don't. I don't know adult medicine, I'm in a subspecialty of pediatrics.* I know his next sentence like my palm.

He moves and blocks my sight-line with the handsome South Asian man in the corner, a flirt who held my hand a few seconds too long when we were introduced. His prune colored eyes studied my face then, as if he were using a microscope on tissue. I told him I'd been to India in the mid-'90s. We talked of New Delhi's air pollution, of Ranthambore National Park's tigers before he moved to a younger woman, a blonde. Now he's alone, nursing his drink as though it contains liquid enlightenment.

"So the doctor said I'm ship-shape, perfect health." Dante pats his small belly, pushes out his chest. "But I told him I need Viagra." He laughs too loudly. There's saliva on his tongue. "Do you know if it helps a woman's libido? Francesca doesn't seem to like it anymore."

My eyes tick around the room until I find her, cheeks crimson, eyes glazed wet, cigarette clenched between her lips. She's perched on the overstuffed chair below the faux Tiffany lamp. I am suddenly exhausted; it's not even eight.

We're at the builder's condo. He recently married a retired stewardess. They're both in their sixties, and he's still smitten, beams at her boyishly, calls her his bride. She details parties perfectly as an upscale pedicure. The drinks are correct, there's an artful tray of hors d'oeuvres, and she baked the candy sweetened nuts herself.

"So, do you know if it's true, that Viagra helps a woman, you know—get desire back? Get her fixed?" He slurs the last words.

What was she thinking marrying him? He's short, his teeth are yellow, and she's slim and funny and beautiful.

Did she do it to escape the knot of island below the heel of Italy? Is there any escape?

"Do you know what's wrong with her?" he asks.

I'm speechless as his mouth unfurls more mud before strangers, a sand-filled carpet unrolled in an oriental rug store. It's been years since I've witnessed this kind of behavior, long, alone years.

I read once that love is not a built house, sturdy and strong—it's fragile, an unbuttressed wall that needs to be rebricked, daily. Their young hyperactive son, Louigi, is their mortar. That, and their weekly case of empties, and the smoke, screening them from each other. His wife uses a long, rose-tipped fingernail to remove tobacco strings from her lip. Someone lights another cigarette for her; she focuses on the red tip, eyes almost crossed.

I remember us in Philly. I could never out-argue you in the small of our apartment. Logic coated your tongue and I was obsessed loving you, being your good-wife. We had separate careers in medicine, one of us always on call. There was constant sleep deprivation, rumored infidelities, denied, denied, and then there were final exams, patient admissions. We were short of humor, frequently out of groceries and clean laundry. It was the '6os, home was my job. But in the hollow of your arms, when we lay close, I'd finger your manubrium, the notch below your throat, above your black chest hair, and relax, knowing the marriage was bristled but that we were smart, we'd work it out. I remember how my stomach writhed when we'd explore our "differences," your desires, mine.

It was only in public, in the safety of a jazz club, or the local pizzeria, with your upper classmen friends, that I could tickle your beliefs, stood a chance of being fully heard, even if I didn't win. How could it be now, almost forty years later, that I'm witness to our sick play, only the roles are inverted.

Francesca must be the homefront victor, if Dante has to resort to public humiliation. I see their ugliness, and I'm ashamed of what I did to you. Women wield power now, but everyone in the room looks uneasy. No one makes eye contact; people eat and drink, turn the music up, embarrassed that Dante has stooped to this, to feel manly, maybe just to *feel*.

I am tempted, very tempted, to go upstairs and get my prescription pad. I still have one. I'd write, Rx: *Make love to your wife like you drink and strut—with single minded attention—make her come, until she cries for release. Don't screw her with Viagra epithets in public like a campaign.*

But I don't do a thing. I don't even try to stop him. I regain eye contact with the Indian, who's thanking the host, slipping out the door. I wanted to give him my card, but I nod, bring my hands together below my chin in a namaste, and go back to sipping my water, which has lost its fizz.

I think back to the evening eighteen months after our divorce, when my first boss touched the back of my neck, gently, just below the hairline. I was hanging a basket of surgicals on the machine, snapping two metal prongs into sprockets. It was summer, and twilight had just emptied the sky of lavender. The samples would cycle through a series of alcohol soaks, dehydrating. By morning they'd be solidified in paraffin, ready for the histotechnologist to cut seven millimeter samples, string them open with a small paintbrush, from the water bath to the slides. A cloud of formalin perfumed the air. We had done two frozens together that day, and before the touch, I was reviewing the diagnoses in my mind, my head half way into a nod that, *yes, yes, they had been accurate calls.*

It's so crisp a recollection I'm afraid my head nods now to Dante, as if I agree with his Viagra crack. That night I stopped breathing, prayed my boss would simply withdraw his hand. Had he turned me, he would have seen my hunger, months without you, without any man. And I needed that job. I was single-parenting our three small children. Those years of laundry, home-cooked meals, grocery carts, and all that lovemaking and compromising had not saved us.

And I loved him in a way, my boss. Had for years. I believed it was platonic, until that fingertip caress. His sharp wit, his brilliance as a diagnostician, and his kindness made my professional life fun and challenging and doable. He was a just man, the likes of which I would not find again for years, if ever. The intense work you do with colleagues in medicine uses your best waking hours. There's a kinetic energy and focus that seals camaraderie. Calling a surgeon with the results of a frozen, knowing a child's limb could be amputated, a foot of colon removed, or a silver-fish fragment of brain tumor irradiated, on your word, is terrifying and a rush that's hard to match.

My boss was half Sicilian, but his temper never flared at me. He used it, a controlled ferocity, in intradepartmental battles for money or space, never against people. Once, only, he told me he'd lost it. It was an ongoing dispute with the head of Pediatrics at the University. My boss had said, "Well, you deal with kids all day long. You're a short, little man, of course you think small."

I loved him intellectually, but I wasn't blind. He was handsome, and some part of me wanted him from the get-go. When he traced all seven spinous processes of my cervical vertebrae with his fingers, my entire back ran liquid. I wedged a hip against the lab bench to stay erect, forced my neck not to bend.

We saw the world alike, he and I. We laughed at the pomposity of some surgeons, worked together in the morgue, over the scope, yoked in this calling, trying to save children's lives. He took the beeper when I needed to get to our children's school plays or a soccer tournament. He let me bring them to my office, listless with fever, gave me time off for emergencies.

I could not go on in medicine without him. I could not go out with him. Where would it have led? My job was financial stability for me to raise our, now my, children.

The histotech will arrive at six in the morning, to prepare sections, stain tissues. We will work together tomorrow and for fourteen more years at the double-headed scope, worrying cells, identifying patterns, questioning each other's acuity. I will call surgeons, oncologists, and neonatologists, give them their answers.

Please, please remove your fingers; don't say a word. I have three small children who need to feel safe. Of course I love you. I'm desperate to be wanted again; you can smell it on my skin, there, where you fingers rest, in the curve below my skull.

I pressed the button, the machine settled its load in the first bath, began to gurgle. I shook my head from side to side, a reluctant, sad no.

I am honored, I whispered. I kept the quaver out of my voice, edged it hard as a glass slide. Tears on my chin, his fingers withdrew. My neck was immediately cold. I wanted to soften the rebuff, I wanted to tell him the whole truth, but I didn't. I remained silent, facing the wall. He went off down the dark hallway, joked with two lab techs. By the following week he was dating one, married again in no time. Our relationship stayed professional. As if that evening had never happened. How could it have?

Dante continues to drink. Francesca smokes and sulks, then begins to flirt with two other men. Dante looks at her, and then shouts one last time. "So doc, you're a professional, and a woman, you must know what makes her dry up like that."

She stubs out her cigarette, makes her apologies to the host and hostess. "Time to put Louigi to bed," she says in a strong voice, lightly accented. "*Ciao, ciao*. I had a fine time," she smiles, eyes clear as crystal.

He says, "Kiss Louigi and eat a few chocolates," as she slides by. She shuts the door behind her quietly. He grimaces at her glorious backside, refills his glass with Scotch, moves next to me. He inhales a cigar and whispers so softly I'm not certain I understand. "We have a saying back home," his cloud of scented dark smoke circles my head. "Beware a sweet-toothed woman, her mouth will grow cold with pain." He shakes his head. "She had a helluva appetite for bon-bons when she was young."

She'll be asleep when he returns, or at the computer. I gave her my password a few weeks back, because he had blocked her from his system. By morning his head will throb, his tongue will be furred, only his manhood will sting with tonight's small memories.

I see how cruel my behavior was with you back then. It was my only recourse I thought: to argue my side in public, make you listen. I'd hoped to shame you from straying.

It could be different now; we might work. Your hair's white, recedes at the temples, probably it's sparse on your chest. Your hormones have decreased, even your scent's changed, closer to an old man's. Your voice is half an octave higher. You might let me win on occasion, although there's nothing left to argue.

I've seen you often lately, at our daughter's graduation in Chicago, planning our son's wedding. We shared the hooding ceremony for him last month, on stage together again, as he received his doctor of medicine.

On our son's marriage day, you strode across the empty dance floor, after the couple left. Our son had chosen old Beatles songs for dancing, music from our time. I found a pair of someone's glasses and a lone centerpiece. The bride's parents were in the back room, checking for other unclaimed items.

You'd frowned at me all morning, except when we danced to *When I'm Sixty-Four.* Your latest wife had looked on, thin and lost from the sidelines. Our eldest girl was at the edge of my vision, but you didn't see her. If she could be happy for her brother's joy, I could remain civil a few more minutes. Your stride was heavy and steady, your face stern. I expected you to hit me with the bar bill. I thought to defend myself with karmic behavior, so as not to spoil the day. My feet slid back a few steps, habit as much as fear.

You began. "I want to thank you for making this such a happy occasion. For all your work and the lovely words you spoke at the ceremony. You were wonderful." All right, I may have made that last sentence up. But you kissed me on the mouth. It was chaste; our lips were closed. No one had been there in so long, tears sleeted my vision. You turned, headed to your current wife, back to me, broad and straight. Your hand rose, brushed the corner of your eye.

As sophomores in med school, we took practicums in pathology. Pieces of patients were sliced at angles we weren't used to from anatomy or our limited clinical experience. One station in the practicum sequence was a specimen in a small jar. Every man in the class put his hand in his pocket at that site. When I got there I saw why. The specimen was a testicle; the question was whether it was enlarged by an infiltrate or of normal dimensions. I was incensed, but recently married, and answered correctly. I jotted a note of protest about how unfair the question was for the ten women in our class of 150.

There was another specimen on that exam, a huge fatty mass, fifteen centimeters in diameter, very thinly sliced. It was covered by wrinkled skin, in formaldehyde. I looked for bone, because I was certain it was a tumor, had to decide between lipoma and teratoma. I finally chose the former, and beside my answer was an X, and a scrawl, "Odd that you aced the unfair testicular question, but missed the nipple on this normal breast."

Faith Forces

"He's done it again. My secretary this time, my secretary."

It's after eleven p.m. in Detroit and I think it's the hospital. "Alice, is that you?" I'd recognize her voice anywhere, graveled, deep, inflected. We've known each other more than a quarter century.

She continues, "The land I bought, the horse ranch? He wants that too. I supported him for three years when he quit the law, paid his child support for heaven's sake. Now he's claiming common law, wants half my retirement."

I sit up, turn the light on, wish I still smoked.

"I manage my investments carefully, they're worth over a million now. He's demented, demanding half. My secretary." I hear her suppress a sob.

"This can't be Carl, the depressive who wouldn't commit. He went somewhere for a real estate surveying course last summer, right? Tell me you didn't pay for that too." I sip a glass of water.

"Exactly, my cash, his degree. He finished with honors, now he claims my land is his. I can't go into it all now, but I'm flying to Toronto this weekend to see my aunt. She's ill. Can you come up for a visit? If I stay here one more week, I'll scour the medicine cabinet, find his old Librium, Lithium, something."

"Of course I'll come. I'm on call; I'll switch." It's dreary in the Midwest in November, a change of scene, even Toronto, will be good. It's no brighter than Detroit, the same run-down downtown in the mid-'90s, and cold, bitter north-cold, but I want to see Alice.

"I thought we Canadians were more civilized than this. Your last divorce from that skanky pilot cleaned you out," Alice says, "and I was smug then, thinking the US is the land of litigation, that we're conservative, more careful here. Now look."

I'm tempted to hiss 'hit man' into the receiver, but I take the phone to the kitchen and make chamomile tea, listen for another half hour instead.

The train jerks leaving Windsor, the car's saturated with seedy teens. Rap music grinds the stale air between bodies pierced and tattooed over every centimeter not marred by acne. Toward the back there's a large woman in a formal fall coat and hat, vintage '50s. Her head's in a book, perfect.

"Honey," so softly I'm not sure she's speaking, "pick a seat 'fore you're jolted onto someone."

I slip in beside her. She shakes her head, mutters, "No Lord, I didn't mean here. I got thinkin' and Sunday's sermon. I meant for her to pick some other place."

I take out my writing but she continues, as if she were learning to read, involved as a child, her words burble. "Okay, she's got work. I take back my meanness Lord, just let her let me be. Oh oh, the porter. Well, my ticket's in the back of the seat, easy for him to punch. I'm not going to look up, open one chink for her."

The train rocks and I wonder if she knows I can hear her. I wonder how stable she is. I wonder how Alice is. If she'll fire the secretary. "Yes," I nod to the porter, "coffee please, black. Would you like anything?" I turn to her, "Coffee, tea, fruit?"

"No, nothing. Wait, yes, coffee would be nice. Two sugars, one cream. Thank you."

She stirs her coffee slowly as fields of autumn stubble slide behind her.

"My name's Etta, Etta Walker. Are you taking a course or something?" She points to my work.

"No, it's a short story, only I don't know. I've submitted it ten, fifteen times; nothing but rejects. And you, what are you working on?"

"A sermon."

"Oh, you're a preacher?"

"No, but my sister Nessa was. Had her own congregation, a fine big one in downtown Detroit. She could pray up a storm, Nessa could, one of those Ella voices. Strong. Strong convictions too, steady household, one man, one son, one daughter. All fine. No drugs. No jail.

"Me, I've been through a number of men, some good, some bad. Six kids, three daughters, all turned out fine. Only Darnelle…" Her voice dries, hardens. "I'm on the train to visit her today. And Sunday, when I get back home, I've got to preach to my sister's congregation. I sore miss her. Best friend for years. After Mama died we grew close. I think before that she was always mad at me for something. For running with too many men, for having to take money from them, from welfare. Well, you can't just raise babies on bread and water. Six before I got my implant." She folds her hands over her book and papers.

I break my cookie, and even though it's chocolate chip, offer her the larger half. Mother would be proud.

"No, no thanks," she says. "Not that I didn't work; I was a medical stenographer, still am. Pay's good and I can do it on my own schedule. And you, what do you do? Just write?"

"No, I'm a pediatric pathologist. Writing's more like a dream. I'd love to try it full time, but. Well, anyway, I'm going to see a close friend in Toronto, a colleague, who's having a tough time. A man."

"Yeah, don't I know." She blows on her coffee before raising it to her lips. "I'm telling you, at some point it came to me, better off alone. My place is small, been in the family for years, far back as my great-grandmother. Course it was always a rental before. She was active in the underground, my great grandmother. That's right, quilt messages, the whole bit. Got herself to downtown Windsor, turned right around and began helping others. Our family's got history in Windsor.

"A few years back, well, more like two dozen when I get to countin,' an uncle of mine was mayor. Two terms. Did a lot of good things for the city. Brought in gambling. Brought in money. People clambering all over him about increasing crime rate, bringing in bad elements. Bad elements hell, we're step-sister of Detroit, crack capitol of the USA. We got all their evil pollution, skips right across the river."

She looks out the window where cloud shadows darken the fields. "Sure do miss Nessa. You have any brothers or sisters?"

"One sister, she lives in Miami. She's a lot younger and, well, we've always lived far apart as adults. We've grown closer now that she's caring for Dad, talk at least once a week. Tell me about your sister."

"The pride of the family, we talk every day, used to. Especially these last years when we were alone, the children grown and gone. Her husband passed, my Henry left, what was that, well, ten years ago. So long without a man you forget what it was you needed him for. Anyway, one of us would take the bus and visit. I'd go to her church on a Sunday and hear her preach, stay to supper. Then one day, just like that, she stops calling. I took the two buses across the river and knew by the no lights on, what it was."

She shakes her head, I pat her hand on the arm rest, the tears fall anyway.

"I know how sore it feels. My mother died last March. It's like somebody yanked a tooth and there's nothing more important than sticking your tongue into that huge socket."

She takes out a man's handkerchief and blows her nose. "Her congregation invited me to speak this Sunday in honor of her. A year already. So I need to do this." She taps the papers on her lap, stuffs the hanky back into her purse, adjusts her glasses.

Sheet lightning dances through the windows. It backlights her salmon felt hat with its pheasant feathers. The storm begins in earnest, rain erasing the drab farm fields that surround naked clapboard houses, Southern Ontario.

"Is that your story, *Garlic*? My granny, the same one, believed garlic healed folks."

"I've heard that. Tell me about your grandmother and then I'll leave you alone, I promise. The underground railroad's a history we just never got in the '50s, we were so unconscious."

"I remembered her when I was trying for my building. I'd sit across the street from it, pull my lunch out and imagine her, pressing cotton pillowcases and sheets, laying them in the closet of her mistress. I thought how her back would've ached, leaning into the hearth for those heavy irons, how she'd get them hot enough to make the cotton smell sweet and sticky, just short of scorch. And her mother before her, bent almost at right angles, picking cotton, balls of white fluff in the same master's field. How it was advancement to move into the house. And her boldness, she told me about it when I was little, how she slipped between those very sheets once, when her mistress was visiting kin. She used that courage to flee. And now here I am, traveling north on a railroad to Darnelle, scared to death." She drains her coffee, stretches her hand, "Story looks short, could I read it?"

"Of course," I say. She wiggles out of her coat, drapes it around her shoulders, and I hand her the piece, pull out a medical journal. The erratic bass of the teen music contrasts the steady thrum of rain on the window.

"Pretty good," she smiles at me above her glasses. "We have small presses in Canada print just these sorts of pieces. In fact my daughter, a different daughter, is a literary agent. She's supposed to take care of my cat, Percival, this weekend, only she's so resentful. That girl, she's okay until she gets men troubles, then she turns on everyone. Daughters can be difficult."

"I know, I have two."

"Do you have other stories?"

"Yes, and a novel."

"If you have a card or something, I'll tell Sassanah for sure." Then, softer, "All right, there's the good deed Lord, now my sermon."

The porter moves through the car again, makes the teens take their feet off the seats, turn their music down. When he reaches us, he pours fresh coffee.

"Nessa was a force, especially when I was trying for my building. She kept saying, pray, girl, pray. He will hear you. I'm not so long on faith, especially now with Darnelle. On the other hand, I got my mission."

"Mission?"

"It's not what you're thinking, not a conversion scheme. It's an arts center in downtown Windsor, for city kids to dance and sing, to paint. Keeps them off the street. It's multicultural. We have inner city Chinese, Vietnamese, white, black, we've got 'em all. My grandson, Celleste's son, runs it. His Mama was none too glad havin' him, so by the time he was five or so, she sent him to me to raise. Well I could see he's smart, so I sent him to college and he came home after four years with an art major. Nothin' to do with that. But here now, it's turned perfect. He's the director, teaches art. We have other instructors to teach dance and poetry. I help out with the singing.

"You know, this is going to sound strange, but through all the planning and dreaming and wanting phases, I talked everything over, out loud, with my cat. Talked with Nessa too, of course. But that Percival habit got so bad, my kids say I still talk out loud, when I'm thinkin' to myself."

The teens go in and out of the restroom. When they return, they reek of tobacco.

"Darnelle started smoking when she was thirteen, fourteen. She'd sneak it outside, thought I couldn't smell. She's the eldest. Forty-three, five children. Her youngest's only four." Etta shakes her head. The music gets loud again, the bass vibrates up through our seats, into us.

"Do you want to talk about her?"

She shakes her head, no.

"Percival sounds like what I need. It gets lonely sometimes. Detroit's a new city for me. I spent my adult life in Denver, so my friends are thousands of miles away, my kids live back East. My job's good, my partner's terrific, and writing's my new passion, exciting and everything, but sometimes, I don't know. When the kids are little, there's too much to do, no time to think. And now, there's all this time." My pen draws small spirals, like a helical virus, across the page.

"I know. My grandmother must've been around this age when someone teased her about not using the telephone. 'I have my reasons and my own ways,' she said. Now I wish I'd asked what they were, her reasons. She was one strong-minded woman. She'd stack her back so straight if anyone challenged her, you could almost see her grow. Sometimes I think she used up the family willpower."

The rain thickens like soup, changes to slush, then snow. We're rocked rhythmically along the tracks. She takes out a stick of gum, offers me one.

"Tell me about your school. How did you get the building."

"Three years of lunches across the street from that place, sitting on the stoop. I ate tuna fish sandwiches muggy Detroit River summers, chilblain autumns, gray springs. Some days it was too cold, and I just huddled inside my winter coat, passed by, nodding, praying for deliverance. A sign went up finally and I wanted to run to a phone immediately, but I knew better. Even though it was February and bitter, I said a long, careful, 'Thank you, Lord.'

"My hand trembled so I could hardly dial. The owner answered and we talked. He knew my uncle, the Mayor I was telling you about. He says what a gent Willie was, all he'd done for downtown business. He'd lower the price, seeing I'm a relative of Willie's. I had $7,000 saved, just-in-case-money. With Darnelle's medical bills now, that seems puny. Lowered was still impossible: $150,000.

"All right," I say, "it's in your hands Lord. And to him, 'Thank you very much.' I hung up, feeling mighty low."

I lean back and she turns fully toward me, the coat slips from her shoulders.

"Here's the thing though, I didn't give up, partly because of Nessa. I kept passing the building every noon, praying. Talked it over at night with Percival, while he groomed himself.

"Three months later the man called me. 'It's May, there haven't been any bids,' he said to set my mind to rest. Then he asked if I'm kin to Theodore and Esma Walker."

"They were my great-grandfolks, organized the underground into Ontario. 'Well,' he says, 'that's how my folks

got here. That railway time, now that'd been somethin'
to live through.'

"I told him then about my dream, about the center for
kids, that it'd be givin' back to the people that kept me
in spirit all those years I sang clubs, worked odd jobs,
learned to type. Maybe that touched something, because
he whittled the price to half. Still, way too much."

She clears her throat, asks if I'll watch her things, and
we take turns going to the restroom. The conversation
shifts then, as it often does with women, moves to love.
Etta begins with Henry.

"That was some man. Handsome, brilliant on the sax,
had his own band, seven records, two gold. When he had
gigs, he kept me and the children in fine style. Early years
I sang with him. But mama raised me right, I kept a job
the whole time, squirreled money away to buy that little
house, free and clear. Sure, we had our falling-outs over
the years, strayed a bit, but he was on the road a lot. We
both had strong natures."

She turns her head to the pane. "One day, after the
children are grown and married, fifteen years and countin', whoosh, he runs off again. *Nevermore*, some line from
a high school poem clicks in my head. Sure, those lonely
blues hit around 11:30 some Saturday nights. Most weeks
though, hot baths, a good book, Percival, and phone calls
with the children satisfy. Oh my, but when he was good,
he was mm, mmm."

"I know what you mean. I stayed years after my second
husband became bad, abusive. I don't know why, but my
body still misses him. My fingers remember his face, the
scar along his chin, how his muscles moved beneath his
shirt, reaching for me. My friend Alice, the one I'm going to see, helped me through that divorce, took me he-
licopter skiing in the Bugaboos. The snow there was like
confectioner's sugar, sweet and fine like the beginning. I
don't know what happens, what makes it go bad. It ended
cold and flat as a penny on a rail."

Long thin fingers adjust her hat. "Every once in a while
Henry calls to see if I've changed my mind. He lives in
Missouri now, says the weather's good for his rheumatism.
Says he fishes, plays gigs, has a good time. That he misses

me, why don't I come down? But I have my life here. Sure, the cold and ice get me down, but I don't have that many needs anymore, and I sure don't have that man craving. I don't know what happened to it, just up and left. Still, it's nice when he hauls himself up, visits. He takes me out, brings me flowers and fish. We cook good meals together, always could. It's hard to cook for yourself. Well, you just don't. It sure does the old body good to put on nice underthings, be appreciated." She strokes her forearms, shakes her head, "You know, each loss shrinks the sides of your life, like it's your own coffin you're whittling."

She polishes her glasses with her scarf and looks down the car to the teens who have paired off now, flirting, kissing. "My sister's gone, ten years after Henry, and now Darnelle." She sighs, "I haven't recovered from Nessa yet, but with her at least, it was her right timing. Now Darnelle, how am I supposed to be? What can I tell her children? She has leukemia; just had a bone marrow transplant. It's a long shot. She's in reverse isolation. I come up every weekend, put my arms through those sleeves, my fingers into too tight, rubbery gloves, and hold her. And, Lord help me, lie. I tell her how much better she looks each time I visit, even though there's less and less of her. I relieve her husband and kids a little. They spend weekdays and nights."

I recap the pen, push my glasses up on my head. "What kind of leukemia?"

"I can't remember the exact name, mycologenus or something."

"Myelogenous, yes. It must be acute at her age."

"Do you know about it? What's the prognosis after the new marrow? I get the impression it's terrible, looking at her, but the doctors won't say. Then too, we're afraid to ask."

"I don't know much about adult diseases. I do pathology, but for children. I started in pediatrics as an intern, and took care of children with leukemia then. That was before transplants, before doctors told adults, much less children, the truth."

"Little children with cancer. Oh."

"I cared for one young boy, Robby, all freckles and carrot-colored hair, so lonely and scared one night, I just crawled into bed with him at two a.m. Against all rules."

She nods her head yes, folds her hands over the damp pages.

"He asked about death then and I said, 'Robby I don't honestly know."

"He was only five, but smart. 'Dr. R, is it going to hurt? How much? A finger prick owee, or bad-bad, like a bone marrow?' I snuggled him tight then, and he continued with questions no one else let him utter. 'How come Mom and Dad shush me all the time when I try and ask?'"

"'Maybe,' I said, 'because your parents are scared themselves. They love you a lot. They're very sad you're sick, so sad they don't want to talk about dying.'"

"Robby pulled away a little then, it was a skinny child's bed, and he sat against the distant bars, right below the window. A Denver night sky held a sliver of waning moon; clouds scuttled across its surface as he stared at me, crossed his arms, waited for some honest adult answer. I made it up.

"'No one can really say if death hurts, Robby, because nobody comes back. That could mean it isn't so bad. Maybe it's just quiet and safe, maybe even fun, so dead people just forget. Like when you go to an amusement park,' I said, reaching for his hands, holding them in mine, maintaining steady eye contact. 'Maybe you have such a great time you forget, like at Elitches' on the Tilt-A-Whirl, when you don't remember your pet turtle, or your best friend.' I think I half believed it myself. Something worked though, because after half an hour of more questions and answers, he laid back down. I held him until his thin body relaxed against mine, and we slept like that until the nurses found us the next morning, luckily before rounds."

"He smiled the next week like we hadn't seen in months."

"Darnelle's so weak now, nothing makes her smile."

She puts her hands over her mouth and I reach around and embrace her as best I can. The countryside blurs by faster, yellow-tan ground lightly dusted with snow, and a heavy charcoal sky. It's a long time before either of us breathes again.

"I don't know whether Darnelle'll make it, but if she has your grandmother's willpower, and yours, there's reason to hope. Doctors get smarter by the hour."

She reaches a hand over her shoulder and rubs between her scapulas. Her back straightens, and lengthens by half an inch. She will not shuffle into that hospital room, bent over. "You know, when I went through that back-and-forth time, wanting that building, unable to afford it, I prayed everyday. Nessa and Percival helped, but I sat alone with my sandwich and spoke to Him. I'm not sayin' prayers are for everyone," she looks right at me, "but I asked for that building and I got it."

Her throat constricts and I see her work to swallow. "Now I'm not so sure I didn't use it up on the wrong thing." She closes her eyes, rubs her forehead, adjusts her hat. "No, the mission's doin' a whole lot of good. The first year we had it, volunteers helped get it functional. My grandson was there everyday, plastering, painting, and we both scrubbed those nasty toilets.

"I still eat lunch from a paper sack at the juncture of McVale and Jackson, only inside now, in a chair, discussing programs. I never enter without thanks.

"So here's what you do, if this is any example," she looks over her glasses at my manuscript.

Oh, a recipe.

"Do your dream."

And I think how in a way this entire desire could be a sin, wasting twenty-seven, almost thirty years' experience. Last month I was called in for a frozen section on a tumor in an infant's foot. It was a low grade, fibrous tumor, rare, but the surgeon was smart and aggressive. We'd had a number like this in Denver, so I insisted he get margins that were free of suspicious cells. I kept freezing the tissue edges, staining and studying slides for hours. The baby was six months old, and by midnight, the orthopedist did an AK, an above-the-knee amputation. I drove home knowing that if I hadn't had so much experience, the baby would have had his leg, but then he would've needed more surgeries fast, or he would've died.

The snow's thick and cottony behind her, a sedative for the eye.

"I'm not sure leaving medicine is right," I say. "It drains me, the politics, conferences, and the autopsies are physically difficult, terrible these last years, my hands," I hold them out, "arthritis. It's getting worse, fast. My doctor wants me to have my thumbs fused, surgery, on my hands. They're my livelihood." I shake my head. "Scares the bejesus out of me. Oh, I'm sorry."

I sigh, stare at my fingers. "Conferences with the parents are the worst. When I write I feel alive. But, I'm a good pathologist, I've spent my life establishing this career. I'm not a quitter."

Etta turns in her seat, her dark-circled eyes brim, "Stop wrestling the wrong walls, you're gonna use yourself all up. You'll die someday, darlin', we all will. You're scared to leave your profession, the respect you've worked for. And you can't see your way in writing. You're worried it's nothing but a late-life fantasy. You've forgotten hunger, poverty. You'll remember soon enough. You've also forgotten joy. And magic, and rest after accomplishment." Darnelle's disease may have burned her hope, but it hasn't iced her heart. She taps my wrist. "Jump girl, just jump."

I embrace Alice long and close before I tell her about Etta.

It's still snowing as we ascend the CN tower, swaying more than fourteen hundred feet above the city which whitens as a profusion of clouds bank the panoramic windows. We get soup and lattés and the waitress tells us Niagara Falls is there, where we're looking, easily visible on clear days. All that pounding water, frenzied and etherized into drops of mist. We finish and go to the deck level, with its glass floor so many stories up, that people, mufflered and hurrying through traffic, are smaller than ball bearings. We're both afraid of heights. Alice is usually timid, but today she winks and says, "Fears are the antennae of a personality. They should be rubbed regularly, to remind us we're alive, while we're here."

Then she suggests we walk the transparent floor. I turn to face her, inch backward a centimeter at a time, commandeering her river green eyes, cupping her hands, saying, "Yes, yes, you can," until we are both safe on the other side.

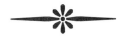

I attend a writing conference in Santa Barbara with a lot of muckety-mucks. I'm in way over my head. My teacher's work is so amazing I'd give an arm to write that well, not just a hand. As I walk to class the first day, there's a pickup in the parking lot with an oversized, side mirror, a block before the conference. I ate a poppy-seed roll for breakfast, and when I get nervous I don't make enough saliva, so I get to the mirror, spread my lips, and pick out black bits, little seeds of halitosis. I pull my sunglasses on top of my head, check the circles under my eyes, fluff my bangs, hold the lipstick tube up when, from the corner of my eye, I see him, behind the wheel. There's so much glare from the morning sun, I'm uncertain. There are two reflected mansions and a man. Is he real? I'm stressed, maybe I'm making him up. But then, he tips his hat and laughs 'til his head lolls back, looks like it might fall off.

L.A. Territory

Listen very carefully, I'm going to tell you how I got my agent. Well, how I *almost* nabbed her.

It was the Santa Barbara's Writer's Conference, snazzy, upscale, summer of '96. A lot of big hitters, author of *Chicken Soup for the Soul*, actors looking for fresh material, fogy editors, passé posers from New York publishing, promoting software, expensive edits to delete adjectives and adverbs, like I didn't know. Then there was Jarine, power woman; a presence, as they say in the business. She entered to hushed recognition; people actually parted for her. When she swept past, the floor moved like unset Jell-O.

She's not the sort of person you'd be drawn to immediately, not the one you'd choose as a seat mate, especially if your plane's stranded on the tarmac. She eats space. And caged like that, she would flow into you, usurping your arm rest, taking up all the foot room, finally invading your head. She dominates every conversation. It's actually a tiny squealing voice, considering her frame, two octaves higher than expected. When she's enthusiastic, she's loud, in that singular way show business people are. Even in her subdued register, her voice grates, a quality reminiscent of my first exposure to Chinese opera.

Listening to her spin twin orbits of self-promotion and gossip that evening, I wondered if she ever sold writers. Publishers and producers probably buy, just to get her out of their offices.

"Now listen Warren, you really do need a piece of this. It's perfect for you, your name's all over the script. An older talent, a notorious Don Juan ages, falls for an unknown starlet. She bears his child, bears the semi-scorn of the public, the jealousy of other starlets; gets him to wed her, something no one's been able to do for thirty, forty years. And then she develops her own talent, which is brilliant. Ten carat. And he, well he disintegrates under the pressure."

I edge close, his response is sotto.

"I don't know Jarine, there's limited appeal for a castralto, even in this era of liberation. Besides, how can you pitch me something like this? I told you I want a renaissance, not a burial."

She waltzes him over to the corner with the food where she holds court, her pied-piper salespitch, *I can make you a star* shines in her smile. She punctuates sentences with Joyce Carol Oats, Alice Walker, Judith Krantz, as though she owned these literary darlings. Occasionally she'll stop, not for breath, but to put something new in her mouth.

"Well Warren, by the time I've located themes you like, well hon, we're none of us are growing younger..." She thrusts a sheaf of papers at him and moves to the bar. "Read it," she calls, at a good eighty decibels, "get back to me. Soon."

She leans over for her drink and her huge purse slips off her shoulder, a sloppy capacious bag. I make a silent prayer it's not a metaphor for her private anatomy.

I sidle between people and chairs, one hand sweat-stuck to my manuscript. I reach up and pinch my earlobe like I'm checking an earring, a trick the school-nurse taught me in fifth grade as she scraped shale from my scabbed knee, an injury from running too fast, trying to get the goal. The pinch distracts me from what I'm about to do, stalking her as she grazes the *hors d'oeuvres*. I collect a plate of paté, crackers, and three over-decorated *petite fours*.

"Ms. Valentine," I hear my own voice scale up, until I'm terrified she'll register mockery. Or worse, confuse it for hysteria. It's third grade and it's my turn in the spelling bee. I know antidisestablishmentarianism. It's been three whole minutes and she continues to call on everyone else. Mrs. Valentine, oh Mrs. Valentine.

"Ms. Valentine, would you care for some?"

She adjusts her glasses slowly, runs her powdery tongue over the perfect fuchsia bow of her upper lip. Just above the white picket caps. Her hand is a millimeter from her mouth, holding a Ritz cracker piled high with crab salad. Her pupils constrict at me, then dilate as she places the entire surprise inside.

I try to puff out a bit, hike my shoulders taller, a greater prairie chicken in April mating plumage, preening at the lecht.

She sniffs more than sees my offering. Finally she focuses on my face, utters a muffled, "Yes," accompanied by a small spray of orange cracker dust.

"Ms. Valentine, I've heard you're the best agent in the business. I have this terrific novel. I'm enrolled in the YMCA writer's workshop in Detroit, and my teacher suggested I contact you. Now, lucky me, here you are. He thinks this is a lot like early Virginia Woolf. I was wondering if....if...I wonder if I could leave it...I mean..." and in a perfect parry, I push the damp pages toward her midsection. A finesse my fencing instructor would applaud, but I worry that my left hand, with the plate, has lifted toward the *en garde* position. I withdraw the manuscript, extend the plate, as her pink cat tongue runs around the outer edges of her lips, laps her incisors voluptuously.

"Who *are* you?"

"Here, have some lobster paté; it's delicious. In fact have the whole plate." I hand it to her and almost crush my manuscript.

It's fourth grade gym class; Mrs. Norace has us still marching. It's been half an hour and all the answers for girl's basketball rules, carefully written on my sneaker soles, are gone. I'm going to fail gym. It's not like I'm doing so well in the other classes. But gym's really embarrassing. I can't do cartwheels, and when I play hoops after school, it's with boys. I don't even know these sissy half-court rules or how long the extra foul time is because we're girls and aren't strong.

"I'm a writer, a serious writer. And a physician. My work is dark, but I've won some awards."

"Well, Doctor whatever-your-name, I'm sorry, I'm not accepting unsolicited manuscripts." She licks each finger with its painted extension carefully, as though a morsel might be missed.

"Sorry," she says, looks at the empty plate.

"Well, I thought on the strength of Sol Stein's recommendation, you might...just a few pages. Let me tell you a little of the story. It's about a young woman who has just lost the love of her life."

She hisses, "I do *not* take unsolicited manuscripts. Not if you were Susan Sontag. And face it, Virginia Woolf, Joan Didion, passé. Sure, they may be taught in colleges, but at home, people read for entertainment, not education. If it's funny, Norah Ephron-funny, maybe, just maybe."

"Well, but that's not the full story, I mean there's romance, and ironic humor. This young woman finds the love of her life in fossils, washed ashore on a beach where she's recovering from being jilted." By an agent.

"Atlantis then, are you going to use the Greek isles?"

"Well, no, I wasn't, but that's an interesting suggestion." It's gym again. "Times up. Put your pencils down."

What am I doing? She's known because she gives great con-artist. This isn't the kind of person I want to finger my words. I reach for my earlobe one last time as she stuffs three great wrinkled olives into her mouth. I certainly hope they have pits.

"Please," it's a sigh, more than a request. I can feel my knees buckle as I struggle through A-N-T-I-D-I-S-E- and because I stutter, a double E weeds me out. The teacher's rimless glasses reflect the light, so I can't see disappointment or disgust, but the horizontal slash of her lips curls down, just before she raps her ruler on the desk. "Now class, let's not make fun."

Her eyes glaze over, content with Greek olive flesh. She reaches across the table for a frog's leg. Who catered this anyway? The pouch under her arm opens and I slip my manuscript in. I mingle half an hour longer, walk back to my hotel. I don't eat much the next two days. I check the mail slot in the lobby four times a day.

Finally, the day the conference ends, I receive the manuscript. No note, just a scrawl across the first page. "This didn't sweep me away...Sorry, J."

Well, of course not, Jarine, I'm a writer, not a gale force wind.

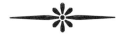

I have a number of great female friends who don't do therapy. They sedate themselves with sex or shopping or housework. I have to say though, they're as well adjusted as anyone. And it's not because the world has treated them with kid gloves. They act normal, rarely confide private torments, unfixable at the most profound level, in my experience anyway.

One has a habit that should catch on. She scrapes her hand hard across her forehead, like swiping a chalkboard clean after school, clasps fingers over her thumb into a fist. Then she flings it open, hurls the invisible contents, unhappy thoughts, anger, disgust, a grudge—away. Just like that.

WEAVE

"I think those chemicals ruined her hair, made it fall out, don't you? Maybe she absorbed the dyes, those bleaches and glues, all those years, that's possible, isn't it?" The February sun's furiously bright in the sere blue Denver sky. I look at Carole's sister outside the church where the air's warm and still, ridiculous for February. Chinooks blew all night.

"No," I say, "it was genetic, her problem."

Her sister's skin blanches ash and she continues. "I bet you didn't know she had the same color hair as you. Nowhere near as much though. Golly she loved those plaitings, extensions, whatever they're called. She had to have them twine all that fake yellow acrylic into her few stray stalks. We were all towheads as girls you know; only she had to stay blonde."

"This isn't my color anymore either," I say. "My hair's almost white now."

She shades her eyes with the back of her hand, introduces me, "This is Carole's writer-friend, Mother." There's Carole's familiar face, only smaller, crinkled. Her mother offers a knotted hand, "What a shame Carole can't be here, she'd be visiting with everyone. That girl could talk, couldn't she? You ever get a word in edgewise?"

"Of course, we took turns. Writers, we all talk too much. Talked."

"Good grief, that girl blabbed everything. Did she tell intimate things about us, the way she told us about you? I hope not." She stares unblinking until I raise my own palm against the unrelenting light. Heat spirals from my black dress, up my neck to my cheeks, even my eyes burn.

"What did she say?" My voice squeaks; it's so dry.

"Oh, that your daughters, you know, you'd cheat on them. You'd promise you'd never see your ex again, that pilot fellow, because your girls were so set against him. But then, love's a hard thing, isn't it?" She winks. "You'd tell your daughters you were going to a medical convention, a friend's wedding, but really, you'd sneak off with him to Aspen or Hawaii, somewhere." She pinches my arm and I jump. I remember now, Carole's mother, the mirror story, the storm, the way she blossomed into sexuality after Carole's dad died.

"You should do like Mother," Carole once said over the phone. "She's got three lovers in her retirement community alone, and she's in her seventies. Two others fly there to visit. She has no intention of marrying again, but they don't know that. She never lets them stay the night. It's the longing to belong somewhere that gets them. They dote on her. They want to have rights too, but Mother's willful," Carole laughed.

I reach to pat her mother's arm, but she turns, spine erect, and walks gingerly into the church, down the aisle. Alone. She slips in beside Carole's husband and daughter, who's folded almost in two. Carole predicted this.

"Lucky for you," she'd said, "your girls will have each other, when we're...no longer here. And bad as my sisters are, we'll have each other when Mother goes. But my Maureen will have no one. Well her husband; but what is that really?"

Carole had high blood pressure since forever, for decades. Then her heart went bad; as in transplant-candidate-bad. Lucky in a way, that I knew the system from the inside, a pathologist. I weaned her from lawsuits because Carole's problems were complex, and she needed someone who'd think well, wouldn't back away because she'd filed claims against colleagues. The initial physician did screw up, gave her anti-hypertensive drugs that damaged her heart, put her into mild failure. She was angry with three different cardiologists, and she hated her original primary care doctor. She claimed physicians, even the women, ignored middle-aged, female patients, dismissed her complaints of chest pain, disregarded her demands to participate in her medical management plan. "Arrogant, over-educated assholes, the whole lot of them," she'd said. "Oh, but you're different," she added quickly. We both knew I wasn't.

She started the mirror story once, about her mother as a child, how they'd had such bad storms back in the dust bowl days in Texas, that lightning often hit houses. "Even as an adult, mother hid herself and us girls under the bed in a storm. We're not talking hurricanes or tornadoes here," Carole said, "just regular rain. Mother was something."

I said my great-grandmother had done the same kinds of things, forbid the use of electric appliances in a storm, wouldn't let us run the tap, or hold scissors. "Wives tales," I'd said.

But Carole said, "No, not true." Then she looked out the restaurant window as big flakes of snow wafted down, and she got very nervous. She hated to drive in bad weather, so we got the check right then, and left.

She went for more cardiac studies, which revealed more things wrong, until she finally found a university cardiologist who encouraged her to participate; recognized it was her life, her heart, after all. He explained what he was thinking before he ordered invasive tests, detailed how they would contribute to her care. He laid out the consequences of doing nothing, Carole's preferred fall-back position.

As her heart problems got redefined, my life broke like a dropped mirror, shiny splinters, years of bad luck. I got rheumatoid arthritis, wasn't able to work the bone saw or wedge the ribs apart. Even fine-tuning the microscope hurt like hell. Then my husband, Lamar, my midlife-starburst lover, grew cold, focused on money, became abusive. There were weeks, months even, when I lived in fear, my health deteriorating in synchrony with his personality changes. He refused therapy, drugs, or talk. A fighter pilot, Lamar never needed help. A year later I was diagnosed with uterine cancer, more advanced than anyone imagined. After radical surgery, I did divorce, an arid place at fifty.

I moved to the Midwest and worked way more than half-time, for half-pay. I hated to leave my heart-home, Colorado, rife with friends and sky. Carole and I continued our friendship, continued reading for each other. She read my stories fast, got them back to me, but I was greedy, put off critiquing her manuscripts so I could produce more of my own.

Carole and her husband, who also has a bad heart (straightforward coronary artery disease), moved to New Mexico, away from the cold and snow. He took early retirement to reduce stress. It was months before she realized they'd settled into a different nettle, a swarm of her relatives. They nested near her two time-sapping sisters, her aging mother. She called often, to find out how I was doing, to bray about her sisters stopping by all the time, without warning, just as she had the house under control, was through procrastinating for the day, had finally approached her computer. She almost sang about the nights though, how her new home spread stars through the backyard, reminded her of East Texas. She was beginning to write fresh again, stories of when she was a girl.

She sent me one about her mother's childhood, about the storm when lightning entered an upstairs bedroom in the middle of night, spun straight through the window to the iron bed her grandmother slept in. Carole never knew her maternal grandmother, felt it was a loss, that her mother's mother would have been a comfort. She was writing toward that, how her grandmother's sudden death stalked her own mother's youth, molded her mother's mothering; impacted Carole's own parenting of Maureen. A sort of biblical story, visited through generations, with a feminist twist.

When she called, she complained about the low level of cardiac care in Las Cruces, and about her hair. "No one knows how to do weaves this far south. I need a sophisticated salon to not look bald." Once or twice she started in on her husband, Ray, but lightly, since I was alone again. "Retirement's a testy space," she said. "Two of us at home all day, he gets in my writing hair when I'm on a roll, still in my robe at four p.m., smoking."

A few months after the Las Cruces move, Carole enrolled in grad school. They seized her talent for what it was, quirky, original, mature. Then her daughter in Denver got pregnant, married, and the travel back and forth wore Carole thin. She stopped wearing makeup, spent all her spare time on-line, or reading, told me she rarely looked in the mirror anymore. "What for?" she said. "Unless one of my sisters is stopping by, all I see is chicken feet skin around my neck, big black circles beneath my eyes that won't go away. Some days, if I squint, I swear there's a faint blue cast to my skin, like people without enough oxygen. Then I remember we're almost sea level here, so that's crazy. Next run to Denver though, I'm going back to see my university cardiologist again."

We filled the distance with letters and phone conversations, but our timing was off. Carole could talk up a storm. She wrote late afternoons and nights, while I wrestled words early. I promised myself not to answer the phone when I was writing, but broke my word again and again. Occasionally it was a sweet surprise, not a bill collector, not the hospital, not my ex. It was her voice, dark chocolate. She still had that light, East Texas twang, with a hitched rasp. We ate hours with our insecurities. Are all women this age jittery, or only writers? I'd mantra to myself as she'd begin, *Listen. Don't talk, just listen. And don't try to match her woes, because really, you can't. Your cancer's in remission, maybe cured. And sore joints? For God's sake, she needs a new heart.* When I joshed her out of the blues, her laugh was cut short too often by a cough. Cigarettes I hoped, or a side effect of her blood pressure medication, not heart failure, please.

She returned to Denver in '95 and we both entered illness essays to *New Letters*, won honorable mentions, hers almost published.

Her heart weakened; she tired. Her baby granddaughter revived her. I returned for the holidays and we met for lunch, crushed each other so tightly, I felt her ribs. We talked through five attempts of the waitress to get our orders. When the check came, our hands met above it, over the table, fingers twined, and we left them locked a full minute.

Her granddaughter's first birthday came and went, and the time spent with her was precious, more important than writing or figuring out what to do about her condition. Carole's heart kept beating. There was indecision and teasing in her voice, "You know these doctors, even the ones who mean well, they just don't know what they're doing."

"Oh some do," I said. "Some have more experience."

"Nah," she said. "They push you though study after study. They don't care about the cost, or the inconvenience, or the pain even. They just want to publish their papers, get their grants. You know, when they did that damned angiogram, it was like they shot liquid Napalm up my groin. It burned my belly right into my chest. Goddamn it hurt."

I'd never heard anyone describe a heart cath before. Of course my patients were silent.

After the New Year I returned to Detroit, struggled with a new word processing system at work. Carole logged onto the Net. There were few women on-line that early; she found virtual space seductive, an ageless place to flirt, suggested I try electronic dating. She scrapped her wonderful Texas short stories, her novel, and started a book for women on the Net, a "how-to" manual, stressing personal safety. She fiddled with the project, got an editor interested, then got distracted with medical data about heart disease in women, how rarely it was recognized, how often misdiagnosed. How women are never given equal opportunity for transplants. "Did you know," she yelled as though the connection weren't working, "women don't even have the same symptoms as men? We get dizzy or sick to our stomachs, spend sleepless nights, break into a cold sweat. Gadzooks, I'm always sweating anyway these days. Makes you just want to spit, that no one ever told us."

Her doctor at Colorado Health Sciences Center ordered a new test, discovered holes between her ventricles. I said, "Ohmygod, a fenestrated VSD. That's a rare anomaly. It's congenital." I'd posted five in thirty years of baby autopsies. I laced my fingers together, phone wedged by my ear, and described the criss-crossing of fetal cardiac muscles as they build the septum, the wall between the pumping chambers. I told her if that muscle grows incompletely during intrauterine life, it leaves a meshwork of fine, pinpoint spaces, like a sieve. "See," I said, "lawsuits wouldn't have made a difference." We both knew nobody knew what would make a difference.

This man reviewed her x-rays carefully; several physicians in two states had seen them many times; he'd studied them before. Now he noticed spinal scoliosis. And a month later, in a dark auditorium at a medical meeting in Chicago, his lightbulb electrified: Marfan's Syndrome. Carole was tall, hid her curved back under loose, blousy tops, and rolled her cuffs, so the extraordinary length of her arms was camouflaged too.

I'd measured arm spans on infants since 1969, when I began pediatric pathology training. I recorded the length of stretched flaccid arms, fingertip to opposite fingertip, then compared that to the infant's height. If the arms were longer, it was suggestive of, like severe scoliosis, the disease that had plagued Abraham Lincoln. Long gracile fingers were another characteristic, like hers laced over mine at the restaurant, clinically, arachnodactyly, spider-like digits; but I hadn't been thinking.

Still, I should have known. I'd lectured on Marfan's at an international genetic conference in Sicily years before. I showed slides of the skin histology, black elastin fibers splintered at bizarre angles in the dermis, background tissue counterstained fuchsia. I contrasted those changes with normal fibers, lined parallel to the surface, making the skin springy, able to snap back after tugging. In Marfan's disease, tension on the skin, stretches it like taffy. The patients often have bleeding problems too, the elastin and collagen in the walls of their blood vessels are fragile.

Some develop clotting abnormalities. I ended that talk with electron microscopic slides, abnormal cross links in the fibers magnified thirty to fifty-thousand times. An irritable Belgian physician interrupted. "Our pathologists studied the same problem, doctor. They used identical methods; but we could not verify your results." He had refuted every presenter all morning.

I took a deep breath, smiled directly at him and said, "Send your blocks to Denver. I'm sure we can demonstrate these same changes in your samples." I rarely have a comeback like that, even Lamar was happy for me. The crowd broke professional reserve, hooted and laughed and applauded. I had a white silk blouse on, no jacket because it was too hot. The applause unleashed my first hot flash. By the time I returned to my seat, my blouse was skin-stuck, all anatomy evident, and my face as vermilion as my slides.

"Oh god Carole, what does he suggest you do now?"

"Well, for one, we need to get Maureen tested." She spoke slowly, "I'll keep you posted."

A month later she called again. "I found a surgeon on the Internet in Texas," mouthing her home-state like a sacred lozenge. "He operates only on Marfan patients, wants me to come to Houston for an evaluation. But you know, I just don't know. Mother went all that way to Dallas for her hip, but it meant the whole family had to stay in motels, and what an expense. We had to take time off too. My sisters, of course they don't work, so what would they know, they didn't mind one bit, all that Dallas shopping. Ye gads, that and gossiping's all they're good for."

"I think you should pursue it." I said, a little too loud. "At least send him your studies and x-rays, hear what he has to say." She lit up, sucking loudly so I'd know the silence meant a decision, and not the one I wanted.

"I could live another ten years with this level of energy, my cardiologist told me last month. Hell, I could finish three, four books in that time. And all those Christmases and birthdays with my granddaughter, I'll get to see her through what, third grade? This guy won't promise I'd even survive surgery."

Smoking isn't helping your heart one bit, I wanted to say. But I used the rest of the call to press again, for her to send the Texas doctor her data.

Soon after we spoke my arthritis flared, I needed twelve, fourteen hours of sleep. Despite thirty years of working hard, sick or not, the new level of pain was exquisite. I finally quit, moved back to Denver, practiced as a locum tenuns.

Carole and I drank champagne together when my five year cancer anniversary filed by, and again when her granddaughter learned to say *Nana*.

"Has that Texas Marfan expert given you his opinion yet?" I asked at one of our lunches.

"Hell no," she slapped her hand on the table so loudly, people in the next booth jumped. "We e-mailed for awhile, she said, but I won't go there, not this fall. I can't miss the leaves turning. Besides, my granddaughter visits every Sunday, all day. I don't think the insurance will pay for an out-of-state consultation, let alone surgery in Texas.

"Anyway, what does he know? They're talking angioplasty now. Something about clogged coronaries. All these years, and some of why my heart's failing is because of atherosclerosis. I tell you," she said, lighting up, exhaling through her nose, like that was still cool, "the more studies they do, the worse it gets."

"You're right," I said, "I don't know what's right, and he may not either. But if all he does is Marfan's, don't you think..." She raised her hand for the waitress, cut her eyes away from me, scanned the room like a trapped animal. I fell silent. After all the delays, the new complication of clogged coronaries, even the skilled Texas surgeon was unlikely to be completely successful.

Carole ordered cinnamon swirl ice cream and looked at me, "There's no guarantee."

I looked out the window at the soft farmer's rain as distant thunderheads stacked, huge and blue-gray. Carole saw them too. "I never finished the story about the storm, the mirror part, did I? Mother was just a little thing, four or five and she said for years she thought the lightning struck because her dad was downstairs that night, didn't protect their mother. Anyway, Mother once said she might have had a problem with men because of that, until after menopause." Carole laughed, then coughed hard. She looked back out at the rain and whistled as spectacular lightning danced above the dark mountains.

"The thing was," Carole added another spoonful of sugar to her ice tea and stirred, "they all heard this fierce noise, way louder than close-in thunder. Mother called the sound fierce. Her folks had one of those crackled old mirrors over the dresser, you know the kind you can never get a full look at yourself, you sort of see pieces. Mother said she smelled something like fire when she got to the room, to her mother's bedroom. It smelled to high heavens." Carole finished her ice cream, licked the spoon. "She held hands with her sisters, and they went in together and there was their mama, dead. Electrocuted, I guess. Her Daddy flew up the steps, pushed the girls back and that's when they saw it. The mirror. Blank. Clean as plate glass. As if, not only had their mother died, but everybody sort of vanished that night. She never did believe her father when he tried to explain, he knew some science you see, that the lightning had deiodized or ionized or something the silver backing on the mirror.

"I'm planning on finishing that piece soon as this heart thing's under control." Carole smiled, spread her long fingers wide, then fluffed her hair away from her skull. "Mother said it was a hard bunch of facts to square for a little girl. She'd put her hands up to her face that night, so even though she couldn't see herself, she could feel she was still there. But she always held mirrors were bad luck." Carole winked, "I'm of an age now, I'd have to agree."

Carole put off angioplasty until it became imperative. They sedated her this time. The procedure went smoothly, bought her another year, but she worried a lot, about the holes, about constantly needing something else done to a heart that still beat a little wild, like it belonged to a far younger woman.

After the service, Carole's mother guides her taffy-haired great-granddaughter over to me. "Carole only half paid attention when we visited, because well, you know, she couldn't wait to get back to her computer, she needed to be typing all the time. She'd grown beyond us. I still have her stories, everything she ever wrote," she stops. "But that's all."

The little girl screams as though she understands, "Nana, Nana," she calls. And her mother, your daughter, appears, scoops her child to her chest. Three sets of dark eyes snap at me, softened by tears, and identical pale wheat lashes.

The funeral's hard, hard earth, still winter, a mother at her daughter's grave. Your mother whispers, "She only had a high school education. She wanted to go to college, she really did. But then she up and fell in love, went running into marriage. She was so happy to get into the master's program in Las Cruces, we were all surprised, no college at all." Your mother shakes her head and I remember how vague you'd been about education, an early marriage, a pain filled time. A miscarriage, you'd said, little Rose, you in your early twenties, young wife, isolated from your family in East Texas, your husband an oil geologist, gone a lot. But you were so prolifically read, and such a damned good writer, no one but you cared about degrees.

We return to the house. I pace the living room, amazed at how your mother's holding up. She says, hospitable smile seamed in place, "If only she'd done this sooner, like I urged her."

Your sister adds, "Carole should've listened to us, should've done this years ago." But years ago it was a heart transplant for hypertension. Years ago they didn't recognize the holes in the ventricles, and the clogged arteries. And still, you might've thrown the blood clot.

Without the full story, physicians would've sewn a new heart to bad tissue, to that aorta, a root of fraying collagen. That union would have split and gnarled with each heartbeat, would not have held the stitching. It would've been like weaving woolen cord into cotton candy, sticky and insubstantial.

Your mother's talking to someone else now, but she sees me, and raises her voice. "You know phone conversations can be wearing, no matter how close a friend. They take a toll on a body. My Carole talked too much, so we worked it out. One call in the morning at seven, no, make that nine a.m.; one each evening." I think she says this to ease my mind, because I didn't return your last call. But how could she know that? I'm in a new apartment, my fifteenth in ten years. It's a shared house, a young tattooed mother lives upstairs with her toddler. The daughter totters to the French doors that separate our spaces each morning. She arrives as I begin at the computer, her breath fogs the small panes, and she calls me until I get up and open the door. I offer her animal crackers and a small cup of milk. Some mornings we share an apple, thinly sliced. I'm here a month, a month and a half before your surgery, which I didn't even know you'd scheduled.

All the mirrors in your home are covered today, folded sheets or pillowcases. My great-grandmother did that too at a wake, so the angel of death wouldn't get confused, grab someone before their time, because their reflection was so sparkly. I move to the kitchen, drawn by your husband's smoke. I quit years ago, but I love that smell.

"Eight hours repairing the holes," Ray says, scotch neat in one hand. "Stitched two new valves in place, a Teflon aortic root, reamed out her coronaries again."

He walks around, cigarette dangling from his other hand, still talking to no one in particular. "She was bruised, so swollen up, but recovering. She dangled her feet. She was cracking jokes for Chrissake. Vain," he adds. "She wouldn't let me see her until she put her makeup on, covered her hair with some fool kerchief, like a cowgirl. And jeans, she asked me to bring her jeans."

Your name's at the top of a list of people I intended to call. Tonight I replay my messages and there you are, a nervous giggle, a swallowed cough, *Where are you? I don't want to lose you, lose track of you. Don't you know grownups don't play musical homes? At our age they grow deep tangled roots.*

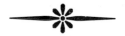

The first time my rheumatologist suggested hand surgery was in 1996, and I stormed out of her office in Detroit, appalled. All she'd said was, "It's time for us to discuss thumb and wrist reconstruction. Think use, not appearance, not the limits you've adjusted to." I felt like some ugly, gnarled finger was pointing at me, like the hand of God expelling Eve, as I limped down the hall, away from her experience and advice. Several surgeries and almost ten years later, I understand what she meant. The pain and lack of dexterity are humbling and humiliating. I have two very short thumbs now, and four wrist bones missing on each side. My palm dermatoglyphics, my lifeline, and the circumferences of a glass I can hold, are all different. My friend Alice called right before my first surgery. "Think," she said, "you'll be able to cook again, maybe sew, crochet even. And, wipe yourself."

Relish

My Aunt Mazie used to nod at aging couples on Myrtle Avenue in Brooklyn, and say, *As God made 'em, he matched 'em.* I could see the resemblance, even at four. I never stayed with a husband long enough to merge that way, although when I loved, I loved with every cell in my body, every single molecule.

I've had more staying power with dogs, or maybe they're inherently more adherent. My Airedale lived fourteen years; my first marriage lasted only ten. The puppy was four weeks old when the children and I brought her home. Actually, we took her to Golden Gate State Park first, in the foothills west of Denver. We stopped for Happy Meals and hamburgers with all the fixings, and picnicked and hiked late that Friday, until the moon rose. The pup didn't have papers. Her father was a famous sire, but his owner got greedy when the litter was large and healthy, demanded more money from the young woman who bred the mother, who had her own great bloodlines. I had no intention of showing her, didn't need the confetti. And I hate bullies. This was a few years after my first husband left, before my second moved in.

The children got to vote on the puppy: I was running a mini-democracy. We sat in the breeder's backyard and watched eight litter-mates frolic for an hour before we chose. The children had already picked the name, Relish. Their father, Michael, ate everything with homemade relish, hamburgers, fries, mashed potatoes, eggs, toast, salads. It was his grandmother's recipe, which I still make; it's really just fancy catsup, tomato paste, vinegar, garlic, onion, mustard seed, oregano, and I add cumin now. Because their dad loved it, they ate it, even when they were tiny, with immature tastebuds. The only food Michael didn't glop it on was dessert.

I'd consulted a vet beforehand, who advised against the friendly, randy males because they were harder to train, she'd said.

We lived in a funkier neighborhood than when I'd been married. People sat on their front porches after dinner, used dogs as alarms. The house had a huge backyard, plenty of play space, and an old, fenced rectangle of dark soil, a World War II victory garden.

My therapist thought gardening would help me out of my post-divorce depression, an almost leveling, extended time of self-pity and rage. Ordinary chores were insurmountable. I managed to go to the hospital everyday, completed my work in pathology, but at home, there were lumps of laundry, sheaves of bills and unanswered letters, and the sink was stacked with crusted dishes and pots. She recommended a series of behavior modification exercises: three cigarettes and a slutty fashion magazine for buying groceries; a collection of short stories and time to read them, after the week's laundry was clean and folded. And for taking the children to the orthodontist: everyone got an ice cream sundae.

The therapist nudged about the garden, we needed an outdoor project, she insisted. There was one small flaw: I hate gardening, resent repetitive tasks, despise weeding, and above all, can't tolerate dirty hands. I rarely read newspapers because the print smears. Even as a child, helping Mother, who at least had a green thumb, I whined as the earth bled through my dungarees, stained my knees. I hated sweat streaking my face, that smell of mud, not to mention its appearance, holds the tang of the last day of menses, rust and detritus. No matter how much I scrubbed after gardening, there were always residual black crescents under my fingernails.

I'd always gotten sulky about Mother's garden, the daily commitment. I didn't hide my feelings, don't, to this day. That might have been a more productive use of therapy, to practice smiling and pretending. Mom saw my frown as I weeded, and said, *You'll see when you grow up: involvement precedes interest.* I thought she was being perverse, or getting things mixed up.

Spring that year still flashes neon in my mind, lovers linked and strolling parks, trees garish in blossom. Suddenly, I was smoking three packs a day, guzzling a six-pack of Coors as if the foam might replace the midnight milky-way Michael and I'd walked under all those years of medical training.

By early July, in Jersey, weeds, aphids and mealy worms seized control of Mother's garden. Her involvement-first crap struck me as totally ludicrous. If involvement's so critical, why am *I* yanking thorns and gray shoots?

I'm an inside-out kind of gal. I care a lot more about the flavor of chicken Cacciatore than how it's presented on a platter. I'm concerned about spaciousness in a kitchen, not if it's got a subzero refrigerator and a trash compactor, but if it will accommodate friends and children and dogs. I'm interested in the content of an apology, the regret in the eyes, the hand held firmly, rather than flowers that scent a room sorrowful.

This was my home, not my parent's, not my husband's, nor my therapist's. But she insisted that if we planted and tended vegetables and flowers as a reconfigured family, we could repair some of the demolition. I was hell-bent on creating new ceremonies; rituals might save us. I had changed; I'd done years of therapy during my marriage.

I paid a local yard man to till and fertilize the soil. The children and I went to a garden store and chose separate crops. My son, Ben, got string beans and corn, because the pictures showed tall plants. He also wanted garlic and scallions for his father's recipe. The girls bought red: radishes, beets, dahlias, tomatoes. I got bib lettuce, a rose bush and kitchen herbs, sage, oregano, basil, thyme, and stiff canvas gloves.

A few weeks later I got a catalogue with an ad for goatskin gloves, *soft and caressing to your hands.* I didn't even check with the therapist, I ordered them. I might grow to like gardening. They were definitely an indulgence, that new, fresh leather smell. Relish found them irresistible too, nuzzled them, tossed them in the air, carried them in her mouth lightly as though they were hers. I like to think she was in love with them because my scent was in them, but it was probably more goat-oriented, instinctual.

I knew even then they were politically incorrect. I was quasi-Buddhist; wore canvas espadrilles all summer. I'd given away the rabbit coat Michael gave me our final Chanukah. The gloves were supple, cream colored, sensuous; I decided to compromise my standards. Besides, I was re-evaluating smoking. The gloves cost as much as three cartons. I needed a reward for even thinking about stopping.

I wore the gloves to train Relish. Well, training's hyperbole. We took long walks the rare weekends the children were with their father. I wore the gloves to protect my hand from the leash. I eased her through early commands. I have a long list of failures in obedience: I never really listened to mother's advice; I disobeyed Dad whenever I could, subsequent beating or not; I never wanted docile children. But that first dog year, I stuck with both tasks, managed a minimally productive garden, a very sweet-tempered, if disobedient, dog.

As solo parent ninety percent of the time, I organized my household, an unnatural act for me, but necessary. Relish recognized gloves-on was either a walk or yard-work. For her, even gardening made me accessible, down on the ground, willing to tumble. She was jealous of the gloves though. If one of the children borrowed them to weed, she got upset.

She was less than a year old when I realized she was no retriever. Relish did little that could be construed as people pleasing. She could fetch the ball, would go once, bring it, bask in praise and attention, maybe chase it again, but the second return was less enthusiastic, a lot slower. By the third time she grew bored. She'd run after the ball, grab it, look back at me, and then either lie down, or cart it to a distant corner of the yard, bury it.

I dug and weeded every other weekend for years, and she'd stand guard beside me. As the children grew and played more and more with friends, there were often just the two of us. Lamar, my second husband, was a pilot, so he swept in and out, flying trips, taking sailing and skiing vacations that my work, or childcare, didn't permit. When he was present, he was intense. He owned a compact virility, a secretive, Jeremiah-Johnson-kind-of-character. His world whirred with a spontaneity that was unbalancing, and seductive. He loved me in a unique, almost lonesome, kind of way. Given my children and career demands, I wasn't threatened by his absences. I habituated to the heat of our desire those first few years; it swallowed all reason.

Winter, house-bound days, Relish entertained herself running up the stairs with her ball, dropping it at the top, tumbling after it again and again. I watched her from the kitchen window in the evenings. She'd toss a toy or a bone in the air, catch it, run around, throw it again. Fetching to please me or the children happened only if that was what she'd intended all along.

Relish loved my children fiercely, never growled or interfered when neighborhood kids rough-housed. She was even-tempered with strangers, except my ex. Everytime Michael came to get the children, a sporadic, unscheduled event, she'd bare her teeth and bark in a frenzied way. If he'd made arrangements, I'd have left her in the backyard, but he refused to adhere to agreements. *Lawyers' rules,* he snarled, then recited his little sentence. *It's my right to see the children when I want, not my responsibility.* The way he said it reminded me of mother's mantra about involvement, but he insisted it was law.

We had a harpy encounter one autumn; I was trying to get him to pay half the children's orthodontia, without lawyers. Almost a foot taller than me, he towered over me in the front hall, pointed his finger in my face, shouted how he didn't have to. My neck bent back like a child's might if she were studying a tree limb, dangling and charred after a lightning strike. I was losing the argument, losing money, losing. Relish came downstairs beside the children with their small suitcases, and Michael backed up quickly, opened the door, exited, shouted from the sidewalk, "Call me."

One of my associates at the hospital was a wildlife biologist turned electron microscopist. The man knew animals. He recommended against hiring a dog trainer, said if only I fed and groomed Relish as a pup, she'd know I was alpha. He was right. Relish was mine through gardens of vegetables and flowers, backpacking trips with Lamar, day-hikes and vacations at the YMCA camp in Estes Park with the children, through two homes and ten bulb-burying autumns. During migrations of the children to summer camp, then college, and finally, to other cities and careers, my second husband tried to seduce her with lamb-bones and tough-play, but she remained loyal.

When it was only the two of us hiking, I shared cheese, fruit, even garden fresh tomatoes. I always brought old, holey towels in the car for her to defrost on in winter, to unclog spring mud, to sop stream water in summer. We'd head off early, a steaming mug of coffee, great road tapes. I'd bring a jug of water for me on the trail; she'd lap hers from streams, or eat snow. I cross-country skied a lot those years, the children on the ski train to Winter Park, Relish and I in the mountains, alone. As she aged, she tired late afternoons and sneak-sat on the tails of my skis, which by then were improperly waxed anyway, too sticky. It often took me half an hour to figure out why I was working so hard. There are entire mountain parks, swaths of Colorado, I no longer return to without her.

Relish had one main idiosyncrasy: her paws. She rarely used them for harsh tasks like other dogs, never for digging. She refused to shake hands. The slightest pressure on a paw made her wince and whine, as if they were tender tentacles. Her snout was her tool of multiple use. She dug holes with it, buried balls, upended boxes or garbage cans, nudged at firmly shut doors, detected infidelity, as odor, long before I became conscious of another cheat.

Lamar was a peculiar man, at home in the wilderness, emotionally stingy, given to showy excesses. For Chanukah our first year he gave me a Lauren polo coat, which I still wear thirty years later, a classic. Another year he gave me a tennis bracelet, all the rage, but I neither played tennis nor wanted politically-tainted diamonds. The final extravagance was an Alpha, red, convertible. The hitch was, he never changed the title, so when we divorced, he owned five vehicles, four homes, all theoretically in love, in both our names...but the deeds revealed no emotional attachment.

Thinking back on it, I might've considered a desert garden when Lamar moved in. It would've required less attention. I could have planted prickly pears, creosote, brittle-bush, even a giant saguaro, whose interior becomes hollow in age, the shell serving as way-station for woodpeckers and rattlesnakes. Lamar frequently met famous people in first class on trips who invited him to sexy-sounding, upscale adventures. Early in our relationship, a famous New York artist asked him for a long weekend to watch his transplanted saguaro bloom. This kind of desert amaryllis needs fifteen years to store enough food to blossom, right before it dies. My love was awakened at three a.m. by his host when the blossom began to peel open and Lamar joined the artist on his bed. No touching, he said. I loved him so much then, I believed him.

When he and I hiked, it was always more vigorous than Relish and I alone, or when I took the children. One September we trekked five days in Desolation Canyon, Utah, along the totally dry Nine Mile Creek. Relish frolicked in the desert while I sweated under a heavy, water-laden pack. There were occasional puddles we purified for her.

For the most part the earth was like menopause, scorching and suddenly arid. The vistas of layered canyons, maroon, caramel, cinnamon, olive, taupe, compensated for the rigor. We saw, but could never climb to, high, secluded granary caves along the creek-bed. I tried not to complain too much. We arose at dawn, hiked all day until four-thirty, when I lobbied for a campsite. For Lamar, the locale had to be perfect: spectacular view, sequestered, although we never saw another person, and adjacent to an overhanging rock ledge in case bad weather hit in the middle of the night. By day four, Relish and I would've welcomed a downpour, manna.

Lamar was ever-alpha, first up, making Ovaltine or Pero, never coffee. Some Mormon traits clung. The final night camping, I was beyond exhaustion, and he was *still* looking for the right place. It was close to seven when I saw a lonely gnarled juniper on a ridge. It felt like three weeks before I reached it, threw my pack down, and said, like Brigham centuries earlier, *this is the place.* But it wasn't. I lay down and watched the sky empty of cerise, then salmon, and turn that heavenly shade of ice-gray, just before night. My legs quivered for an hour. I really couldn't imagine standing on them again; but he continued, compass in hand, sighting mountains, treading over ridges which looked wrong to me, toward the sunset. We'd entered from the east; not where he was heading, a lifetime ago. His impossibly accurate sense of direction was wrong. We parked over there, I pointed, to where the moon would rise. Relish padded ceaselessly between us, back to the tree, ahead to him, until he vanished, and the evening star appeared. Eventually he returned, grabbed my pack, cajoled me with promises of a great dinner and back-country lovemaking. I came to his camp.

In the morning I was certain he was heading further from the jeep. The lot was in the opposite direction; I'd been great in the woods back east. Two hours grumbling how wrong he was, before the yellow hood shone on the horizon. Without this man I would've died of thirst.

There were trips to Paris, tours of the wine country, luxurious, alcohol-blurred. Roadside cafés with extraordinary meals, aromatic and unrated by Michelin. Once, for lunch, we had radishes and sweet butter as an appetizer, a carafe of local wine, combinations I would never have experimented with: exquisite. We stayed at four star hermitages and castles, drove curving backroads past griege-vineyards, and rouged hillsides. There was a gray-white region, clay soil where locals insisted the bones of wild horses had been scattered centuries earlier, herded over cliffs by Cro-Magnons. The crispness of the local wine was unique, maybe a touch of ash. I missed Relish sleeping with us, she would've loved the land. I saw a bustard in one of the vineyards, realized Dr. Seuss hadn't made everything up. We made bets in France, whoever or-

dered the weirdest meal and finished it would earn sexual
favors, on demand, for the rest of the trip. I ordered an-
dolettes, a sausage stuffed with intestines. The meat was
served under sauce, of course, but it was stingingly bitter.
Bile coated my tongue; and I needed a carafe of red wine
to finish the "delicacy." He had one bite, laughed and said
I didn't have to; but I'm not one to call uncle.

There were other times we were happy too, and then
it aged. Just not like fine wine. He became angry, more
and more easily, grew impatient with my children, con-
sumed with money. I stayed. I loved him, I said. It was
more complicated, we had combined finances, owned a
mansion together, loved the dog. He hadn't changed titles
to the "us" yet. I developed arthritis, ignored it for two
years, then couldn't. It got treatment-demanding bad. I
needed ten hours of sleep a night, then more, plus naps.
Work was a challenge. I brought a sleeping bag and pad to
the office, rested between autopsies and frozen sections.
There were days reading slides, alone in my office, when
just moving them on the microscope stage made me cry.
My knuckles were huge and red. I had a new boss who was
erratic, shaded the truth here and there. At home, my husband lied about our finances, his gambling losses, used
questionable tax deductions. Small corruptions I easily
ignored, but they pitted me anyway.

My friend Alice visited one weekend after a pathology
meeting and we hiked most of Sunday with Relish. We
hadn't seen each other in almost a year, needed catch-up
time, talked relationships, a little medicine. "Carl and I
are linked," she said. "It's our fourth incarnation. I love
his kids. We have issues, it's been six years. We could
never separate, our finances are too mixed. We'd never...
survive." I knew what she meant. She petted Relish continuously on the ride back, even though she had classy
lapdogs at home. With papers.

Lamar wanted us to all watch the Broncos, but Alice
hates football. I thought he'd understand, and he seemed
fine at dinner. But he sulked after she left, I'd excluded
him from the hike, he'd had to watch the game with kids,
meaning my children. I tried broiled salmon with dill cu-

cumber sauce, rare steaks and martini, fresh crab legs; he would not be pacified.

Before things totally disintegrated with Lamar, we took a final back-pack trip to Grays Lake, Idaho in June, to look for re-introduced whooping cranes in the huge breeding flock of Sandhills. The white birds were a head taller, clumped together, but all the cranes clacked their bills as if they were huge wooden spoons smacking hollow logs. They squawked and jumped in feathery balls, fanning their plumage. There was an unconscionable infestation of mosquitoes, food for their chicks. As soon as we got out of the jeep, every surface blackened. The bugs got beneath sunglasses, under hats, up sleeves, and shorts. They coated our eyes, hovered around ears, then zoomed in: ears, noses, mouths. I wanted to camp there anyway; the birds were thick and elegant, but my husband immediately leaped back in the jeep, rolled up the windows, while I shot roll after roll in the swamp of birds. Relish stayed with me, squirming as mosquitoes got in her eyes and nose. She was often conflicted if Lamar and I separated. She was my dog, but he always hiked with liver treats in his pocket. I felt that was cheating, but it worked.

We stopped at Bridger-Teton national forest, western Wyoming. My arthritis was cranky from all the ground sleeping; I walked slowly, needed to catch my breath from pain, but pretended to jot in my journal, reload the camera, adjust the F-stop.

Lamar insisted on one last night camping out. We hiked from ten a.m. until late shadows encroached. The trail narrowed precipitously to half a foothold, partially covered in old, iced snow. The ridge of avalanche-scree sloped several hundred feet down, at a forty degree incline. I was worried about slipping; I was worn out. I knew something was wrong with me, seriously wrong beyond the arthritis, just nothing I could name. I tried to keep up with Lamar, tried to stay balanced. He was far ahead, engrossed in his late day hunt, searching for perfect. Relish loped between us, raced ahead to him, tried for the lead, looked back for me, intent on keeping both of us in view. She returned just as my left foot twisted, slipped. I hollered, grabbed at a clump of sagebrush with gloveless, gray-blue hands. I held air as a volley of small stones accompanied my slide. It was slow motion at the top, accelerated midslope, so I sat down to slow myself, a fanny toboggan. Relish watched from the top, then followed. With four feet, she climbed up easily, slid down again and again. She must have repeated the process six happy times during my single, labored ascent. She loved the rush of the hill, the speed, being out of control.

Lamar heard my yell, came back fast enough to see the end of my fall. Aggravated by the delay, he stood and watched Relish climb up, slide down, and wound up clapping and laughing. That rant aborted. I distinctly remember him asking if I was okay. He still loved me.

The next morning when we got back to the car, Relish had to be lifted in. Lamar hand-fed her bologna sandwiches on soft white bread, bought her milk for two days, until she regained her strength. That was the first time I fantasized about being his dog.

During early courting, Lamar respected my independence, bragged about it to a friend, playing hoops. "She's safe," he said. "No interest in money, this one. A libber. Refused alimony the first time. All she cares about are her kids, and the sick ones at the hospital, tumors, dreadful, depressing. Spends nights reading how to diagnose new tumors, leukemia. Damnedest thing, when all they'll do is die."

Back then, both Relish and Lamar treated me as if I were special. Then he moved in. His jeans and scent stippled our home, boundaries blurred, Relish grew confused as to who was lead-dog. Maybe it was his demand for my attention, or the way he doted on Relish, or how he resented time I spent with my children, or at the hospital, but it started to deteriorate, just a little.

The first summer all the children went to camp for six weeks, I didn't plant vegetables. Instead I made a romantic English-cottage garden, high altitude variant: larkspur, columbine, pink asters, day lilies. Late that summer,

Lamar started flying to the Far East. There were weeks I was alone with Relish. That's when she had puppy-regression, "accidents" in the house, chewed the children's clothes, several pathology textbooks.

When Lamar came home from trips that summer, he was hungry, for me, for home cooked meals, more demanding than ever. It reminded me of his mother's story when I first met her, in her Salt Lake City home. She said Lamar had been a terrible baby, didn't nurse, refused the bottle, so skinny by three months, she thought they might lose him. They lived in a mining town then and his father borrowed a neighbor's car, drove fifty miles to the doctor, who said Lamar was starving to death. He said to feed him anything he'd take, cereal, milk, mashed carrots, potatoes. The baby plumped right up. Food was still religion to the man.

The needier he was, the more petting Relish required, more walks, or she dribbled in the house. I missed the children in an aching physical way that left me wilted, and I wondered if her dribbling was her way of crying for them. She gnawed her bone loudly when Lamar wrestled me to bed after dinner. The more I met his demands, the greater hers grew, until I found myself walking the dog alone, late at night. Cheeseman Park in the dark was not smart. Relish marked every few steps those nights, territorial, I thought, or maybe stress-related incontinence, because Lamar was always grabbing me.

She found my gloves again, in a pot with a trowel and a dandelion digger, as he and I lazed in the hammock, reading. I'd just weeded and was sipping iced tea. Lamar had a new Desmond Morris book, blaming mothers for the world's woes; I thumbed through medical journals. Relish clasped the gloves between her paws, brushed her muzzle over them. Maybe in her dog logic, if she had to share so much of me with him, then I, too, had to share. Toward twilight, she tossed the gloves in the air, watched them flutter to the ground, slow and frayed as August butterfly wings.

Lamar's moods swung wildly when the children returned that fall. His hunger for me, flattery at first, became claustrophobic. That winter Relish's leaking worsened; I started taking her to vets. First, urinary tract infections. I collected samples with blood in them, midstream. I'm sure the neighbors thought I was weird. I gave her aggressive antibiotics, took her for more tests, x-rays, dye studies, consultants. Nothing stopped the seepage. Now when she sucked the leather gloves, I let her.

She had bladder cancer. She was only four. The young vet who diagnosed the cancer operated. I stayed in the room. She removed half her bladder, and a perispinal lymph node. I studied the slides, they were filled with dark blue, malignant cells, and inflammation. An immune response, so that even though the node was involved, she had a complete remission.

The veterinary literature on bladder cancer in dogs gave a four-month-survival, tops. In our happiness having her home for what I thought would be a brief parole, I was too permissive, let her romp all over the backyard. Her stitches broke and she developed a urine-peritonitis. Instead of whining or snapping as a human would have, she simply dug a hole with her snout, a large, deep one, while we ate lunch, and heaved her bloated abdomen in. When I found her, she was so lethargic, I rushed her to the vet, Ben cradled her limp head in his lap in the back seat, saying sweet, loving things to her, coaxing her to keep up the work of life.

She made it.

The following year she was still alive, symptom free. Lamar put her on his lap at dinner on the anniversary, fed her a T-bone, rare, which he'd cut into small pieces. But she had a recurrence. The symptoms were easier to recognize. I thought she'd been through enough, but Lamar said, "If she were a child, you'd treat, wouldn't you?" Relish was the only dog to have survived bladder cancer more than five months. The vet was willing, re-operated, removed more bladder, which had restretched by then.

"I took most of the cancer," she said, "and another lymph node." Also positive. She thought there were more nodes. Relish was a gentle, trusting dog. I removed her stitches at home, talked to her, and held her head as the vet inserted the urinary catheter to give her intrabladder thioteppa, an old leukemia drug from the '50s. I soothed her through two years of chemotherapy. I'd talk to her, stroke her head, and she would lay perfectly still, secure.

Alice visited that fall after attending a conference on placentas. We sat outside in November, warm again, Denver's best-kept secret, its stash of sunshine, as Relish romped in the yard. I told her about the tumor's recurrence, what little hope I had, how Lamar was insistent everything be tired.

"Have you done a healing?" Alice asked.

"Oh, I know you believe in reincarnation and all, but I don't know how you can. We're scientists, doctors."

"You never know." Alice elbowed me.

"If I could heal these paws," I held up red, swollen hands with bulging knuckles, "I'd believe. Hell, I'd be eligible for the Nobel."

"Right," Alice said, "but what could it hurt?"

Relish was at the end of chemo. The vet said her last x-ray showed a large, recurrent tumor in her bladder. The sun was fierce that afternoon, as I rolled her, so her belly splayed up. I held skeptical hands over her abdomen, focused my mind to a pinpoint of yellow light on her bladder, visualized horrid purple cells succumbing to sun.

We had tuna fish sandwiches on the back porch, and I shared more of Lamar than I intended; how things should be getting easier with the children grown, but that they may have been our glue. We both had compelling careers, no financial worries, but now time hung ripply between us, petunia petals late season, frayed, losing color, tedious.

I helped the children with SAT preparations, college applications, but I'd always quietly worried about Lamar and me alone. Now Relish was dying, everything in flux. I was terrified, in a superstitious way, of the changes.

Lamar groused that winter at the children sloughing chores, defying control. *Normal,* everyone advised, *they're becoming independent.* Maybe because I'd worked so much when they were younger, I felt their separation like a spade cutting an earthworm, a lethal error, leaving both parts quivering. Lamar said I was being ridiculous, just exaggerated empty nest, but I went back into therapy, anyway, called Alice, often. She understood, spoke of her

stepdaughter at twenty, madly in love. "I could tell her
what not to do, how to save her heart. This yahoo's going
to break it. But what will that help? She's in love, won't
hear a thing."

Relish remained overjoyed each time I came home. At
least someone was. Her physical demands were a comfort
too, walks, nuzzling, regular as a fetal heart. Lub-dub,
feed me, lub, let me out, dub, pet me, lub-dub, nap.

My Aunt Mazie said long time couples do more than
look alike; they borrow clothes, philosophies, laugh at
the same jokes. Even early, some couples mirror, she said.
*She gets pregnant, he eats too much. Constancy's what does
it. Every morning at coffee, at dinner, beside each other on
the sofa, first face at daybreak, they leak into one another.*
She didn't make it sound romantic.

My vet claims there are similar connections between
people and pets. She means beyond the superficial, how
some owners look like their animals. The preppy page-
boy types with their Labs or goldens; the frizzy permed
women sporting poodles; the trendy, with Boucherons and
SharPeis. She says individuals and longtime pets share
a certain humor, she's seen it, and sorrow. "Illnesses?" I
ask, because we've treated children at the hospital, whose
pet died of a tumor the year before they developed theirs.
"Well, of course not," she says. I agree.

A year after Relish's chemotherapy ended, I was diagnosed. Lamar and I were in a bad place when my tests
began. He was gone a lot then, in town for the surgery,
then back in Montana, celebrity chasing, fact-checker for
a Redford film, almost out of our frame. My surgery was
more extensive than Relish's; at least it felt that way. It
was my body. I was super scared. I had uterine cancer, not
bladder, lucky me. But no one, not my children or friends,
not my doctor, certainly not my strong-man husband, let
me speak my fears. They were as afraid as I was, afraid
of losing me, and thought the way to postpone death was
the magic of not naming it. Maybe they were right; I'm
still here.

My entire hospitalization was a drugged cocktail party of chatter interrupting pain, the weather, pain, political events, pain, drugs, blossoms of gossip, pain, nausea, pain. A bouquet. When I got home, Relish was there. She alone was willing to listen, head cocked, ears accepting my terror. She gave me space. I took a long time to heal.

When I recovered from the cancer, I returned to work, but my arthritis worsened. I would be in a credentials meeting and someone would tell a lie about documents or present a competitor physician as unscrupulous and my hands would flare, red as fire. I asked for honesty, but where turf and money are concerned, even physicians who care for children lose all sense. I quit the committee. My secretary was friends with the lady chaplain, suggested I talk with her. "I'm seeing a therapist," I argued, miffed.

"What can it hurt?" My secretary asked. "One visit; no one has to know."

I went into the chapel, I'd been there before. Sometimes I brought a baby down before an autopsy so the grandparents could hold him. I also hid there, hard days with three or more posts, when my spirit melted. I would come and sit, my hands opening on my lap, as if I were doing yoga or expecting a stigmata, some visible punishment.

Chaplain Jane smiled, offered ginger tea, asked if I were to die soon, what my regret would be, besides leaving family and friends. I almost yelled, *writing,* said how the cancer made me recognize the one thing I'd always, always wanted, that I didn't know if I had any ability. That my marriage was disintegrating despite couple-therapy, date-nights, time-outs. We were both efforting heroically to save it. And then, unprofessionally, I wept.

"My hands," I cried, holding out molten maroon mitts. "They hurt all the time. They wake me in the middle of the night. I can't embrace my husband. I can't use the Striker saw any longer. I can't even scissor dissect. Somedays, I cannot put enough pressure on the forceps to pull tissue to see where I'm going. My diener does it all now; I stand and watch, useless. And I'm selfish since my surgery." My head bent low over the teacup.

She put her left hand out between us, and said, "Do you believe in healing hands?"

"Don't be ridiculous, I'm a doctor."

"Put your tea down, put your right hand out, over mine, just don't touch." Her dark brown eyes held mischief, a demi-smile. What the hell. I did what she asked. She floated her right hand, palm down, over the back of my extended hand. I looked up at the clock, 3:50; I had a frozen in half an hour. There was a crucifix, and a shelf of books about grief and prayer.

I read the titles, not a single book spoke to me. I still had to check on the electron microscopy from yesterday's neuroblastoma, finalize the report. What a waste. I looked at my hand, at her hands, and felt the heat rise, not in the room, in my hand. Only the color was draining from it; it was salmon-pink again. I looked back at the clock, five to four.

"Gotta go," I said, and stood. "Thanks for listening. Thanks for your time. Sorry I was belligerent, I'm not long on faith." By the time I got the specimen from the OR, my right hand was normal; I could put a size seven glove on again, move the scalpel like the old days, surely, without scratching the tissue because the pressure hurt too much. My hand worked all night. I diced vegetables and my husband and I made love. The next morning, before nine, I was in her office, my left hand thrust toward her waist.

"Maybe," she said, cradling it in the air between her palms, "maybe the cancer was a wake-up. Maybe you should be doing something else with your life, your work, your home, what you were meant to do."

"No, I've had all this training," I fanned my pale right hand in front of her face, swatting the suggestion aside. "Almost thirty years, diagnosing tumors. I'm good, a good teacher, good bench pathologist, meticulous in the morgue. Surgeons come to watch me dissect. I'm a great diagnostician. I can't. I own a huge home with my husband; I'm almost fifty." My hand fluttered like it was trying to remember if it was the right or left hand of God, you wanted to sit near.

It's summer again, the mid-'90s and I'm in Toledo, divorced a second time. I'm in the hammock Lamar and I shared. My yard's lovely, corn and beans, high, and the tomatoes are plump, blood red. Turns out I'm not so different from Mother after all. There is comfort in habit, tending small green plants. I still wear gloves, still dislike dirt. I've relocated here to work half-time, live quietly, write a little. Baudelaire said, *Make your life orderly and regular, so your writing can be violent and original.* There's a small kitchen garden by the side porch, thyme, chives, rosemary, topped with purple crowns. I planted lavender along the fence; its fragrance frets the air like mountain rain, like Lamar's scent, still in the fibers of the hammock, revived damp evenings. I remember those summers we rocked gently, sipping oaky Rhone, reading. Relish would slide beneath us, brushing, swaying us. She wanted to come up, but that would have disturbed us. I could pull her in now, if not for the arthritis, hers and mine, and if the hammock's threads were less frayed.

Besides, had we brought her up, the reading would have stopped, she'd have inserted between us, like in bed. There was one afternoon she strolled below us and trotted off. Today she finds shade, circles five times, folds herself into her swept bed of grass. That afternoon it was long paragraphs of Margaret Atwood's *In Training*. Lamar read McMurtry's *Leaving Cheyenne*, interrupting me to share what interested him: Wyoming landscape, details of bedrock that pointed to subsurface oil and gas deposits, wildcat speculating. There was a jolt, Relish returned. My soggy cloth gloves lay on the ground. She circled, sniffed them, left. I read two more pages, musing, dozing, then lurched awake. She'd come back and the hammock dipped as he tried to pull her in, sixty plus pounds with one arm. I reached over my side, for counterbalance and cupped my wine, "Damn, I wish I had those old leather gloves."

"What?"

"Goatskin, remember? I trained Relish with them. First indulgence after my divorce."

"I didn't know you owned leather anything, such a purist. Vegetarian. No fur, hell you don't own leather sandals."

"Yes, I know, I'm trying, but this was an earlier me. Those gloves felt like silk. I got them right before I stopped smoking, an early reward. Please don't pick her up and spoil the afternoon. The gloves—the last time I saw them—on the porch. I was going to plant impatiens in that shade, below the hickory, before that bad storm."

My hands began to caress each other, palm over back, massaging the now liver-spotted flesh. It was almost a cellular memory, their malleability, like covering skin with lily petals. I could still smell the cured sweet hide.

Relish returned, her snout filthy with soil, a wad in her mouth.

Lamar saw it first, asked, "What's that, an old bone?"

"No, I think, maybe, nah, couldn't be."

It was matted and muddied and salivary. Two plus years. "Where'd you get that girl? Drop it, good dog."

Definitely a hammock-up trick. I helped her in, leaned on his broad chest, and in a seductive purr, said, "I want the pair sweet Relish, bring Mama the other glove." Then I bit deeply into my apple and put a chunk in her mouth.

I scanned the yard and counted at least a half dozen burial sites, bones and balls, a graveyard. Undisturbed. I kept scanning and saw a patch of fresh earth, a new mound over by the fence, under a bush. I toss the apple core and Relish bounded out of the hammock, ate it, and began to circle the yard, furtively looking back. Secrets.

I squinted into the sky, like I wasn't watching, as she retraced an ancient ceremony, burying time. I shook my head in disbelief, we were both sun saturated and wine dozy, beginning to nod off when she returned. This time her treasure was crusted in heavy brown mulch. What was once delicate cream, scented with animal rheum, now smelled of earth.

Relish ages rapidly in Toledo. It starts with subtleties, a few strands of gray in her saddle, a central refractive crystal in one eye, then the other. Her hearing declines, although that's hard to judge. Airedales are notoriously stubborn; she's never paid attention to commands.

The same year arthritis wallops my knees and hips, the stairs become a challenge for both of us. We rise each morning, stiff-legged and halt-step downstairs; her to yard necessities, me to making coffee. A large hallway mirror reflects our stumbling descent. And we both see it, I catch her eyes smile at me in the mirror more than once. We go to a new local doctor and vet, begin new medications. Our tumors stay in remission. When the barometric pressure falls, my rings no longer fit, my knees grow big and boggy, she's in more pain too. Some days, she doesn't let me touch her.

The second summer in Toledo, Relish stands frozen by the back screen door one night, gazing steadily at the garden. A rabbit. I'd seen several, the lettuce is raided regularly. Relish's vision has deteriorated, but her nose is fine. She lays down, hurrumphing, and watches like a cat, tail twitching spasmodically, head angled this way, then that. She remains suspended, only no rabbit. It takes several minutes to accommodate the moonless dark, but there they are: minute, intermittent fluorescences, a yard of fireflies.

Static's not how I remember Relish. She had as much spitfire as my great aunt. The mettle that made her impervious to training was one of the things that bound us.

A year after my recovery, my incision split open too. I didn't get peritonitis, but the hernia was so large that everytime I laughed, my intestines pouched beneath my belly skin, you could see the peristalsis. It hurt like hell. I stopped laughing. After the hernia repair, my belly was anything but beautiful, and I hoped to be looking at it for a couple dozen more years, so I had a feather tattooed across the incision to remind me that every woman conceals something under her skirt.

Alice visited after that surgery, not to help so much as for company. Alice was a great gardener, so she did fall mulching, laid new bulbs. She suggested I get a new hair color and cut, update my pre-divorce wardrobe, move the outdoor herbs into pots. As her visit wound down, she lingered each morning in her room. I assumed she was meditating or talking with Carl, but she was with Relish. Communing, apparently. "She's a wise old soul," Alice said, then embraced me tightly. "Quite an extraordinary dog; she's been around before."

"You're not saying Relish is reincarnated. From what, a roadrunner?"

Alice laughed. "I know you don't subscribe, but she's a real spirit. Has she ever spoken to you, communicated in any way?"

What a question. From the full professor, author of two texts on placental pathology. But I had an answer.

"Yes. Twice. Once, when Tori left for Belgium. We were hugging on the couch, having some of the chocolate cookies I'd baked for her to take. Dunking them in glasses of milk, when, clear as I'm saying it now, Relish stretched over and said, 'cookie.' It was Tori's and my secret; no one else would ever have believed anyway."

Alice doesn't blink, "The second time?"

"I was going into the hospital for the cancer surgery, it was the night before. The children had flown back, all asleep by then, different time zones and all. I was on the porch sipping my second scotch, neat, enjoying a cigarette. What the hell I thought, looking at the moon. Relish was beside me, stirred a little, stretched her head way out, like a giraffe, and with extraordinary work, you could see the muscles tense in her neck, she said, 'Mama.'"

One thing I've learned with age: some memories should stay buried. Extramarital affairs, a too-close brush with the law, a slow waltz with cancer. The last visit to the vet.

I still can't say her name without choking.

People pressed me with advice, *Replace her right away. A different breed, a puppy will perk you up. She's no longer suffering. Or, it's been weeks, move on, for heaven's sake she was only a dog. Other friends advise no pets, you have no responsibilities now, simplify, travel, go away for long weekends, stay late at work.* Now there's an incentive.

I held her in my arms as the needle entered. I whispered her name over and over, close in her ear. I held the goatskin gloves by her nose, a scent she loved. And as her breath evaporated, I saw her toss the gloves in an Alpine meadow, in very slow motion, pale leather fingers slicing ribbons of columbine-colored sky. She is young again and so are my children, back home and still small, the world of growing and possibility stretches ahead.

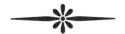

I requested slides from my mother's autopsy to review with a colleague, a neuropathologist and good friend at The Children's Hospital of Michigan, in Detroit. I was trying to be cool, taking brain slides from the box, but my hands shook, many were stuck, and my arthritis in a flare, so he removed them. He also did the steering over the sections that day, pointing out telltale Lewy bodies, overwhelmingly abundant throughout her cortex, especially the frontal lobes. He spent time reassuring me there were no neurotangles, the pathognomonic feature of Alzheimer's.

Late Sentence
A Conversation Mother and I might Have Had

It's eleven p.m., the room shudders against light. Fecal odor fouls the air, strong as a philosophy. An old smell: the living room bassinet, my brother Danny, dying of dysentery while I played with his long fingers, tickled his sunken belly until he laughed out loud. Mother is this whole room, flat white sheets her frame, shapeless as a drop cloth spattered with pain. The IV drips, constant siren. My sister, Deb, sits, bone face collapsing into itself, eyes drift in dream. She senses me before I close the enormous space between us, before Mother's intestines grind again, milking something through, loud as her scolds belled over our playtime, *Come in, wash your hands, don't talk back. Get your father's slippers, do as he says.*

Finally, it takes all this morphine and dying to bring her here, to her knees, her senses, her rightful place. I tried, God in heaven knows I tried, to have her behave, be a dutiful daughter. And to take it easy, too; but even as a child she did everything hard, hard measles, hard headed, bad fights with him. Her sister learned to work him, wormed her way into his heart. Not her. Not that I didn't envy her spirit, but God's witness, I tried to rein her in.

My sister unwraps her lean, six foot frame. Where did she inherit such stature, grandparents from Eastern Europe, Jews with those squat, pear bodies. Mother's mother tall for her day, five five, died in radiology, Mother out to lunch. Her habit playing ostrich, ignoring what Dad performed on us, her vacancy inuring her of evil. The way she'll wind her time down here, waiting for my watch to end, no one by her side, not Dad, who cannot bear to see her, curled around her heart, thin skin parchmented as organdy. No, she'll wait until we all stop waiting, and then, like Danny deposited in that hospital, white as a flash, she'll go.

My name is Dorothy, it's Wednesday, and I don't give a damn who's president. All this fuss when I've nothing to say, not really. Deathbed confessions, passing something on, please. I'm so clotted with drugs, I can barely think. I wanted things to be fairer, she does too. But you know, it doesn't work that way, life. My early marriage ruined by an unwanted pregnancy. Her. And the war. My honeymoon years back home, silent while my parents spoiled her rotten. He was in India, Tahiti, came back changed, full of sex and rage. We moved to Jersey; I lost myself, became his.

My sister whispers, *Oh, thank God you're here.* Mother's smile pretties her face like lace edged slips when we were little. Mother saved all smiles for him. Those blue eyes snapped in daylight, laundry on a line in a stiff breeze, her look let things be possible, like hope.

Our son, born in '47—his death, the worst. That bitter bitter church winter, snow piled high as the roof. A white christening gown for burial, a doll's dress really, on a thread thin body-so pale he glowed lighter than the satin coffin lining. He wasn't baptized, our boy: a Bris. An agreement: the girls, Catholic; the boy, his. Then the priest refused last rites, and I refused the church, then him, a duty in anyone's faith. Then he refused to breathe, my husband did, hospitalized for months: asthma.

My sister drapes herself over me, and I let her. She smells clean: soap. A relief to breathe something besides mother, and my own salt tears. She never knew Danny, born three years after him, but I still love him, cannot recall my own sister's infancy. Blank. All I have of that time's blurred, a thin, blue-swaddled baby, gray skin, green stools. I raised her though, Mother vacant for years, my turn to soothe again. Mascara dribbles weep lines down my sister's cheeks, as we embrace. But it's not her comfort I came for, not really, my guilt needs stifling; I need mother.

My husband and his asthma-drama after Danny: oxygen tents, injections, ambulances. And me, bleeding until I was white, almost dead myself. Subways to Manhattan, to Sloane Kettering, scraping my insides daily like a burned kettle. Then the tube to Jersey City, to visit him, flat and morbid, gasping, until one day, I came early. There, leaning over the nurse's desk, butt exposed through the back of his gown, dick hanging between stick legs, laughing, flirting, dark eyes snapping.

My sister leaves, goes home to her husband; she still has one. Beige walls pulse fluorescent as my watch begins, twentieth century bedside: waiting for the crisis moment, which has no chance of arriving.

I'll hold my son soon, please God. I never meant to trade his soul for peace in that household. All my rage is gone now, years of slow attrition, worn with him. What I let him do to those girls; how will they go on? At least they have each other. I so wanted a sister my whole life, and here now, they have one apiece, don't seem to appreciate it at all. Seems like you can never please everyone. Seems like, God knows, what I've found, you can't please anyone. But who'd believe me speaking up, this late?

My mother was always able to put on lipstick without a mirror. She applied perfect pink or rose or red lips when she was thirty and fifty, even seventy, with her Parkinsonian shake. She'd rest a pinkie on her chin, sweep lip rouge in a semi-circle, holding the tube between two fingers like I held a scalpel or a pen, or years ago, a cigarette. She always made a bow on the upper lip. I watched mesmerized. She said, "If my hand doesn't know where my mouth is by now, well, I'll have extra color on my cheek."

Tremble

Dear Nola,

I wake up and feel it again, in my right hand. It's happened five, maybe seven times the past year: a faint, fuzzy, dissociated tremor. Only this morning I'm in bed, in the light that reigns Taos when I hold my hand out. It really moves. This is more than a premonition or a dream. Yesterday was my birthday; this trip a gift to myself, fifty-seven years, still ticking.

Wasn't it just yesterday we first met, new wives, new mothers, lives bursting with husbands and toddlers, newborns and all that cooking. Hellman and Camus punctuated our conversations, along with Vietnam atrocities, peace protests, potluck picnics.

The last seven years have been a montage of reinvention, relocation, regrets, celibacy. Well, not quite celibacy, and not by my design, but that's a different letter. The flutter continues above the sheets, movement with shadow, as though my right hand were run by a different brain. Immediately I go to the future, uncertain, how long the stretch of aging alone. It terrifies me.

I share your ferocious longing to be intimate again, biting as a live electric wire. I want to see my children more often, visit you regularly. Only the children are adults now, independent, scattered across the country. And you, you're...distant. Our friendship spans decades, more than confidants, closer than blood kin, we are selected sisters.

And I know what it means, the hand. Mother died of Parkinson's. The information will wreck my family. For the first time in forever, I won't tell. I've been ill before, brayed each diagnosis in blind rage, as if speaking the disease might dismantle it. Maybe it was my substitute for prayer, raising complaints so loud the universe might take pity, take it back, make malignant, benign. Then I would have looked silly for carrying on, and gladly. All those protests never changed a single prognosis.

My children, my sister Deb, will be stunned. It's not supposed to be hereditary. Then, they'll shriek personal fears, worried for their own risk. They'll talk with doctors, get on the Internet, weigh genetics, some may pray. All will shiver.

I've looked at this from a thousand angles Nola, and the only upside, which you'll love, is the drug of choice to treat this makes you horny. I went back to the gallery this morning and bought those earrings. I don't need more decorating, God knows, but I need cheering. For awhile I'll be able to get the posts in, secure the backs. I'll wear them until the tremor worsens, until I'm unable to fasten buttons, which will be followed, if Mother's progression was the model, by shrunken handwriting, my signature shriveled and jittered. My voice will wither too, stringy and dry; thoughts will cluster and clump, sentences disconnect.

I'd scream shit, but for the accident three days ago. When I swore then, the small bruised child near the road reacted. She lay on her stomach in the dirt, arms and legs flaccid, as I kneeled by her head, crooning, "You won't die. The ambulance is coming. You're going to be okay. I see your family. They're fine. Don't move, help's coming." I wiped blood and spittle from her cheek, and when I turned my head, I saw a sheeted, smaller sibling lying impossibly still. "Shit," I whispered. Her body contracted. I stroked her cheek again, apologized for my language.

She wheezed, "I have asthma. Make the ambulance take me first. I can't breathe. I'm afraid I'm going to die." I ran to my car, got my inhaler, pumped medicine into her, forcing her airways, at least, to move.

The paramedics arrived in a testosterone blaze, and despite her protests, cut her new blouse up the back, with sterile bandage scissors. We all saw the tire tracks where her flesh was pulverized, saw the broken skin welt, purpling. I saw beyond that, a fragile spinal cord, white, flayed.

The southern Colorado sky was a glorious blue. The soil was shit-brown, which I must've said out loud again, because she grew agitated and I apologized once more. The ambulance attendant told her she'd be fine, in a dry, rehearsed monotone.

She could not move her legs, knew some of her future. I claimed the rest of her mind with chatter so she'd fight. I would have healed her, if I owned enough belief, but all I did was stay, stroke her hair, squeeze her hand, tell her she had years of dancing ahead. The paramedics said it was cord shock, not permanent, although they were meticulous strapping her head into the cradle on the stretcher, to secure her for transport. I insisted they check her head straps again, brace her more tightly, scolded them, *Be careful, go slow, go fast.* Please, let my assessment be wrong.

Just before they moved her, she rasped, "I love you."

"Yes, darling I know," I said. "I love you too."

I miss you Nola. Only once has someone matched your temple-bell laughter, and she was mad with love, saved it for him during their courtship. You were more generous with sounds and food, with your time. Had you not volunteered, again and again on that first call in the morning, to baby-sit my children when I was a resident, I could not have finished my training. My sitter would cancel on the spur of the moment, and you, who loved babies, anybody's babies, saved my profession, let me finish my three years in pathology. Those days were a long, sleepless blur: children, medicine, my husband, cooking, groceries, friends. For you it was home, your daughters, your friends, greedy reading. Your marriage was so solid, you wore it like a shawl you'd woven from wool you'd carded and hand-dyed.

Remember later, my visit with you in Santa Monica? I was at some medical meeting, stayed the weekend to see you play Lily Mortar in *The Children's Hour* at a community theater. You were wonderful. We went to the cast party and I flirted with the director, stopped paying attention to what I was mixing, had several too many. I was so tanked, I fell on our walk home. Damned platform sandals. I ripped the elbow out of the peasant blouse you'd loaned me. Then around three a.m., I got so sick, I missed the toilet. You said no matter, got up and cleaned it, bathed me like a baby.

I feel silly repeating our history in a letter, but I need records. The last long chat we had was right before my hysterectomy.

"Hi honey," you said. I heard your voice smile. "How are you? And his majesty? Happy now that he's got a new throne, I mean home, in Aspen? Tell me about the girls, pardon *moi*, the women. What are they up to? I miss you." I called to wish you luck with your surgery. Of course you're not going to need it.

"Me? I'm still at Fox, still looking for Mr. Right. Bad weeks, Mr. Right-Now. Working with show business people is like toxic tinker toys, they construct ego-castles with smug-rings. If I could harness insecurity here, I could power LA for a century, klieg lights and all."

I asked about Lily and Colette. I didn't want to talk about the surgery, or him. He was hovering, and you picked up on that.

"Later for the girls, us first," you said. "I'm doing a new kind of therapy. I know you've heard this from me before, but she's spectacular. She sent me to a retreat: energy fields, chakras, auras, vintage L.A. I love it. On the couch, in real life, we deal with my mother. I know, I know she's dead already. I'll go to my grave talking about her. But the way I know it's working this time is, when I call my sister, I don't need a drink before, during, and a double, after."

You were hopeful that night, you'd met someone at the retreat, and I wanted to channel your energy. I closed my eyes and the miles dissolved, your arm looped over my shoulder, your armpit bushy in the French style, our brown braids brushed each other's skin. I saw those enormous dark eyes of yours, mahogany circles of passion and a kind of eternal innocence. You laughed, "Let me tell you about Colette and Lily," but your laugh held a little sadness, like brass beginning to oxidize.

I remember your daughters, playmates to my girls. We were only slightly older than they are now, when we met. I'd call, stop by after work, nudge you on a Sunday, *Let's go to the park. Please, make your chocolate mint pie, and I'll bring burgers and salad.* We wandered the tuliped parks, all the children wearing themselves out on the slides and swings. Our research-scientist husbands played tennis or smoked pipes, talked about immune studies on nude mice. We spread blankets on newly sprung grass, ate and talked until the moon came up.

"How's Colette's neck and back?" I asked. She'd been struck by a drunk driver at seventeen, spent most of her senior year in high school in a halo cast. Colette was your baby, conceived in Paris in the '60s, quiet and moody. Delivered during the student protests there, your husband frantic, hailing a cab in his broken French. He earned his post doc in someone's lab while you learned French cuisine, cheap horsemeat and herbs.

"Neck's perfect. Her head aches in the rain. And she is her mother's daughter, doesn't want college. She wants theater."

Colette had your giant eyes, only gray, which grew huge in concentration as she followed her older sister's every nuance. A reservoir of un-American silence. I wonder, and you must've too, if she was some sort of a marriage barometer, her thumb the plug in her no-smile, serious face. A map none of us could read. She loved to be rocked to your lullabies though, sung in French and Yiddish, smooth as the applesauce you made each autumn and canned for December latkes.

"She does stand-up a couple of nights a week. She's terrific," you continued. "Studies costume design, works odd jobs, coffee shops, manicurist, whatever. She's so beautiful, high cheek bones, definitely Irv's. She wears her hair like you used to, long and straight, dark as rum. She lives with me, in the same cramped loft, keeps the rent down, keeps me company."

Colette, a woman. I still see her sucking her thumb while we drank, smoked joints, a mild metallic taste far back on our tongues. She couldn't have known then, none of us did. But six years later you divorced Irv, a year after he got his appointment at Columbia. Both girls grew up with you in a Santa Monica cheap flat. Their Daddy married his lab assistant months after the divorce. Young girl, new start, fresh baby, suburban home, the American dream.

The roadside girl looked a little like Lily when I saw her last, gangly limbs, curls framing a thin face. Accident "helpers" on cell phones ground glass into the shallow soil, which sprawled east to a fuzzy horizon. The child's siblings were scattered across the meadow, blanketed in the stubbled grass. The father crawled gracelessly, his forearms swords, cutting space to get near his children. People crouched over him, tried to wrap his shoulders in blankets too, tried to slow him down, telling him the children were fine, the ambulances were coming, it would be okay.

In the van, in the distance, a green web replaced the windshield. Lines fisted tight enough to pull the sun out of the sky. Inside that metal trap, the mother was caught behind the wheel. And inside her, moving spasmodically, was a six month fetus, head cottoned by amniotic fluid and dark blood. But it was the child who could not move her legs who kept me immobile, keening inside, watching the chaos the same quiet way I studied cells through the microscope. I turned the fine focus and found the hole in the back of the van from which the children had been flung.

Lily was the leader of our children, graceful and quick-tongued hilarious. She helped with the babies sometimes, paraded with us against the Vietnam War.

"Tell me, what's Lily doing? Is she still wearing her hair short and punk-colored? Is she in love?" I whispered the last question, because I was out of practice saying the word, hadn't used it out loud in over a month. He was still eavesdropping.

"Is she doing theater? Should I recognize her name?" She would have graduated from UC San Diego by now, but she'd quit. You called to wail about it at the time, said it was pure spite. And, like my girls, she's grown up guarded. I kept asking questions, hoping he'd get bored and leave.

Your voice caught. "Lily's back East now. She's applied to NYU film school, compliments of Irv." You tap the phone with a glass, as if toasting.

"Merlot," you said. "The small Sonoma vineyard where the retreat was held. It sucks. I mean Lily, the wine's fine. She lives in the city, works as a waitress, has a weight problem, misses me. She won't admit that. If she lived here, the weight would melt off. She never had a problem when I was cooking. And her hair? I have no idea what she looks like anymore. She won't send pictures, won't even call. Her own mother. She's in some kind of shitty therapy. Irv pays for it, and she insists it's the three thousand miles that lets her stay sane and emancipated. Get that, emancipated."

They're our children Nola.

You went to France, remember? Then Denver, far from your Boston roots. I traveled half a continent to rip out my mother's chaining umbilicus. Although, I still missed my Nana's Sunday dinners, roasted garlic chicken, mashed potatoes and gravy, field-cress salad with her sugary dressing.

Remember how we mocked our mothers then, s*mother-mother-love* we used to chant Sunday afternoons, after the obligatory morning calls back East, instead of church. Our eldest daughters both moved East, a direction neither of us deliberately gaze.

East is where the van careened, after colliding with the jeep. It hit a gully that somehow jimmied the back and streamered children across the field. It looked like some farmer had gone mad, sowed damaged human bodies instead of seeds.

The mother must've done some fancy maneuvering to keep the vehicle upright. The paralyzed girl, closest to the road, was probably first ejected, then run over by the jeep, whose driver was dazed and banged up, but basically fine.

The night before my surgery, you kept talking, "To answer your doctor-question, Colette's vertebral fractures have healed in proper alignment," you said. "As to motherly issues, she's definitely out of her halo. Mouthy and defiant. You know the early twenties, me, me, me. She sees a therapist too, but her woman's a genius, encourages her to follow her passion, forget college. Irv's screaming mad about it. I'm not positive either; look how hard it's been for me with no degree. I have to say though, Jewish mother or not, you've got to see her on stage. I mean, when you recover. Let's plan a visit. She's strong and witty, innovative." You swallowed more wine. "Her therapist thinks it's natural she lives with me, healthy. Now your turn, tell me about your girls. Talk. Talk."

"They've grown too, opinionated, too opinionated. Strident and funny. Their humor's so quirky it has to be your influence, all that heroic baby sitting. Some weeks I'm so proud of them, I can see their names in lights. Others, I'm certain there was a delivery-room mix-up. They do things I can't bear to hear about. I wish I still smoked dope."

You laughed, your three-part bubbling harmonic. "Got some great shit at my retreat. I'll save it for your visit. More, tell me more."

"Tori knows just how to get me. First thing she did when she went East, to her father's alma mater, was change her name. Legally. Now that's emancipation."

"I'm so sorry," you said. "What do you call her then?"

"I still call her Tori. But everyone else, even her sister Ariel, calls her Emily. If only she weren't as secretive as Dickinson."

"It's a bitch when they're finding themselves," you said. "Everything's a new betrayal. It makes you almost rethink your own parents. Only our rage was justified, right? Look at how much time and money we've put into therapy, cleaning our psyches so we don't visit those mistakes on our children. But they turn on you anyway. *You didn't hold me enough; you were too intrusive; you never cared, didn't ask.* It doesn't matter, you could be a pure genius at parenting, and all they see is hostility. Or neglect.

"I sent Lily a bumper sticker: *It's never too late to give yourself a happy childhood.* She wouldn't answer my phone calls for two months." You paused, then asked, "What's Tori / Emily doing?"

"Working a donut shop, finishing last semester," I said. "Last Christmas she stopped my heart, said she was thinking about joining the CIA."

You didn't even take a breath. "The thing is, if she's like Lily, she's closed enough to be on their payroll already. Last Chanukah, Colette and I flew to New York. We were at the MOMA when Lily announced, 'You raised us to think for ourselves, Ma. And now that we do, and don't subscribe to your leftist leftovers, you get all cranky.' She said it straight faced, with a ring through that surgeon-perfect nose of hers.

"I never told you what really went down when she left LA. Irv flew her back for some cousin's Bar Mitzvah. Just a long weekend, that's all she'd packed for, and he promised. Of course that was an Irv promise. Once she got there, he screwed with her head until she decided to stay. When I called, Irv wouldn't put her on, said she was afraid. Can you believe it?

"She stayed with him and his doll-wife, five years older than she is, well maybe ten. Colette told me they watched soaps every afternoon, took field trips to Shorthills mall. My sweet Lily made up stories of a tortured childhood, like horror plots for a film class. I mean, I love her and all, don't get me wrong, I just don't know what gets into them, especially firstborns.

"But she learned something from that girl-wife," you added. "Lily's wheedled Irv into footing the bill at NYU, *if* she gets accepted. And her own apartment in the city. I never taught her that kind of manipulation," you sighed. "She should be out here. LA's the place for acting. Come to think of it, she should've had to drive cross-country with two screaming children in a ratty old Volvo, become a character actress in her forties, if she wanted drama. Emancipated my ass."

I wanted to go back to neutral then, to calmer topics before surgery. He'd gone to bed.

"Ever think about the commune we used to discuss when we got stoned?" I asked. "Remember how we'd drive around to find the perfect house in downtown Denver? Both families were going to live together. I wonder how things would've turned out."

"It might have saved us," you said. "I mean, the children, our husbands, maybe we'd have been swingers."

I think back to how we really were then, slim budgets, midriffs floating through pregnancies, believing in possibility. I used to make little deals with God each time I got pregnant, if this child's born healthy, I won't complain about another thing, no matter what.

Dots of color dance across the page. I'm writing to you at Café Taza. There's a plastic bag half-full of water in the archway, fragmenting sunlight.

A tall man passes the table and shadows the letter, now on page five of an oversized legal pad. I flex and open my hand several times, rub it, look up. He's got long blond dreadlocks, ratty jeans and a little boy straddling his hip. Our husbands never parented like today's men. His scent's strong, no deodorant, little soap. His beard is thick and bushy, like Irv's was, a thing I envied, but was afraid to mention, afraid it might be misinterpreted. You both caught something sensuous in Paris, something animal, and that never changed. When I look down again the page is clearly written in a full, firm cursive. I've got time.

I wish you were here with me Nola, not just for your laughter. There are graveyards outside Taos still festooned from Easter, redolent with pink flowers and banners, pictures and tiny pairs of shoes, little clean socks. You'd love it. And the architecture, the way stucco curves around every corner, even the doorways curl feminine. The smallest details are elegant, a cerulean windowsill, weathered wooden shutters, a pot of geraniums. It's the way you accented your apartment. I can still see that fifty-nine cent Target vase with a sprig of lavender in your bathroom, the stretch of white walls in your living room, hung with a single picture, *space to rest the eye*, you said. Our home was plastered with posters, cheaply framed, and a few family snapshots. The most creative thing I ever did was paper our bathroom, floor to ceiling, with medical diplomas.

You asked about Tori on the phone, but I'm thinking further back, thirty years now, to when we signed power of attorney to you and Irv for our children, in case we got jailed at Woodstock West, Saturday's march.

"Remember how we dragged them to peace rallies and feminist protests in backpacks, in strollers, in utero? Well, it took on Ariel," I said, "like a vaccination. She has my curse: a true believer. She led a protest recently against a campus beauty pageant in Boulder. It was a Playboy contest for a coed centerfold. When the doors opened, railing feminists swarmed the auditorium, and a line of male students pirouetted across the stage in string bikinis. She was outraged. She never even laughed. We would have."

The waitress at Café Taza and I have gotten friendly. This afternoon it's just the two of us, as she warns me about dating, "Taosinos," she calls them. "Don't bother about where you'll eat, or what to wear. Don't even worry about small talk. There's always his pickup. Do find out if he has indoor plumbing, before a second date."

I thought she was kidding, but she said the young father with the dreads is one. "Off-gridders. They live in earth-ships out in the desert, semi-buried hovels, dirt-filled tires and bales of hay. Disgusting," she said. "No plumbing, no electricity in most of them, unless they steal onto a line. One wall's windowed for solar, and plants. They need plants, for the oxygen. Those pits are closed tight as a tomb, windows don't even open." She shook her head and went back to wiping tables.

Years ago Ariel and I came down here; she wanted to spend a night in an earth-ship. The eco-tourist version was show-home classy, a moneyed interior with niched couches, burnished mahogany book cases, chips of malachite and lapis set into stuccoed walls.

When the waitress refills my coffee I ask her about the bag of water in the archway, is it hung just to produce rainbows.

"No," she laughs. "An eco-trick against flies. They come up to the bag and see their image magnified into a hundred-fly army. They retreat." I wish we could use a trick like that, simple, cheap, astonishing, to deflect our daughters from danger.

Even those earth-ships weren't as claustrophobic as you sounded, calling from intensive care, the night of Colette's accident. Lamar and I were in the middle of another brutal fight, so I didn't pick up until the fifth ring.

"Colette's in a coma," you sobbed. "Her skull's fractured, she's got three broken vertebrae in her neck." You may have been wheezing, but I was so intent on calming you, on getting details, on checking, long distance, that her care was correct, I didn't notice.

Lily and Irv flew in the next day, stayed until the worst was over. Later you said there were no accusations, no, *had you stayed married, not left New Jersey, there might have been a son.* No, *had you stayed, Colette would have been driving a car, not taking a bus, would have had a metal jacket of protection around her.* There was none of that.

All your Lily and Colette stories kept mixing in my mind that night before surgery. I was scared, kept seeing us younger, the girls tiny, tamable.

"Cancer!" you'd shouted. "I don't believe it. Are you sure? Are they sure?" And then, to distract me, you spoke of on-line dating disasters. The one I remember was young and slick, an Israeli. Six feet tall, sexy as hell, fabulous accent. He had a great hairy chest, you said, and it took months before you pieced things together, figured out he was an arms dealer. And God bless you, horny or not, you dropped him like a scorch.

"Oh, but now Adrian," you said, "from the retreat. Best biceps I've ever felt. Long blond ponytail, slant-blue eyes. The color of hyacinth after you've put iron rods in the soil. And he's hung." You lowered your voice as if my husband were on an extension, then cleared your throat. "I've heard about your no-goodnick, through our daughters. He's a royal prick. You're losing your uterus, so promise me you'll give yourself a gift after the operation. Promise me, you'll at least think about leaving."

I couldn't talk about anything important that night, so you continued. "Funny how we have to pump our daughters to find out the skinny on each other. And sometimes we learn things we'd rather not, about our own daughters from our talks. Life's truths are always gossip."

A week after I got home from the hospital your postcard arrived. It was an eerie photograph of a woman's face, blurred out of focus, the image dissolving. You had redotted the eyes with blue ink and put an enigmatic, Mona Lisa semicircle in red, where the lips would have been. On the back you wrote, *You're going to heal perfectly. I hold you in white light. The universe is protecting you. You'll be fine.*

That's what I told the mother in the van, as more ambulance sirens pounded. People wandered the field mumbling quietly as if they were at a Sunday service. A meadowlark called out its territory every ten minutes. Sirens must have shrieked through your apartment that night Colette was hit by that drunk, a stolen car, around the corner from home.

The van that spun off the highway was a rental, another daughter told me. She sat upright, ten feet away, teepeed in blankets. I spoke to her when I could, her voice ragged, as if she were very old and extremely tired. She told me about the family vacation, the ruins they were supposed to see at Mesa Verda. How the sand at the Great Dunes National Monument had run through her fingers exactly like the beaches back home, like Jamaica. How even Colorado's sky was the same color blue. And then she asked if the rental place would be mad at her mother, because of the wreck.

Once the girl I knelt beside was safe on the stretcher, I hurried to the pregnant mother. Her hair was crusted and darkening, an oxygen mask covered her nose and mouth. Her eyes were wide, desperate. She was being told over and over by the paramedics, Do not move, don't shake your head, at the same time they fired questions about where she hurt, if she could feel her fingers, if the baby was moving. She sat, wedged behind the wheel. The airbag had not deployed. She stared quizzically at the scree that was windshield, as if trying to interpret a message. Her look reminded me of the moose I'd seen years before in Denali. Tori accompanied me on a birding trip after the first divorce. She was only eight, and it was ridiculous to take her out of school like that, but I needed her. She loved the exclusive mothering. Then.

I had bad insomnia, worse in late Alaskan light. We hiked a trail in the park one evening, were still out at eleven p.m. A huge brown hulk stopped, not twenty feet off, flanked by skittish twins. They were as curious as Tori, whom I immediately harnessed in my arms, so she wouldn't provoke them. The ranger warned us about moose being more aggressive than bears, especially with young. I slipped my daughter sideways into the forest, the green thick and hiding. The moose twisted her head, studied me, shook her antlers, collected her twins, then turned around and went back the way she'd come. The musk of her was like strong shitake mushrooms, it stayed with me for days. Tori still won't eat mushrooms, says it's the texture, but I know better. Memory's so fickle.

I elbowed between the paramedics to get close to the mother in the van, touched her shoulder. "I'm a physician," I said. "Your children are all alive, they're going to be okay." Firefighters trundled across the field with a welding torch as her hand shot out and grabbed my arm. Slowly she turned her head and I met her gaze, knowing that to dislodge her body safely, she'd have to believe something, true or not. I spoke the name of each child as the upright sister had recited them to me, told her the details I knew she could bear.

The men carved an archway in the metal to remove her. I don't know how her children are or will be, of course, especially the youngest, who'd been whisked by me beneath a blanket, too quickly for me to check his chest to see if he were breathing. I didn't tell her how her husband crawled over the land like a marine on his belly, used his elbows like crutches, punching the parched dirt, moving to his shattered children. And I didn't say that I was relieved I wasn't driving the jeep. Or that I was silently thank-God-ding my children are grown, can dance.

Your voice always sang of the '60s, Nola. Trippy days of irreverence when we'd congregate in someone's home, eat on the floor, pass a J, strum guitars, children in and out of laps. We believed principles would preserve us. There's no hanging out like that now. Everyone's busy, eats out, surfs the net, doing, going, moving, gone. When I was a little girl, Mother and I lived at Nana's, a bosomy nest of women. Nana's sisters were close, and every Saturday morning without fail, they'd arrive with fresh crumb cake or jelly donuts, drink coffee with yellow, satiny cream. They talked about how the war was going, especially in the Pacific, where Dad was. Aunt Mazie called it the Pacific Theater.

You left Irv on an impulse about theater. Courageous, after one acting class. You told me you knew then, knew he would never understand, that you just had to try. His voice cracked when he called me, frantic, confused, asking who the guy was. I was divorced by then myself, didn't know what to say. I knew you weren't having an affair, we were always in touch back then, I was certain. "No lover, Irv, I swear." I said it three times.

You'd simply wed too young, bore your children before you had time to fashion yourself. We all knew that, but you carried it so well, no one believed you lived half-fulfilled. And if any of us had suggested that to you, you would've protested, *That's so bourgeois*. But there it was: one bright spring day, this time of year, your garden mulched, pale green crocus fronds splintered the soil, and you split. For LA and a career you imagined would fulfill you, like a mystic seeks God. You drove west with your daughters, your high-school diploma, a typing award, one hundred fifty words a minute, and hope. You did fourteen hour days on the road, you later told me, buzzing right through Denver, not stopping for sleep, a visit, a breath of mile-high air.

You temped, took acting classes, did commercials, got your studio card, raised the girls on zest and ingenuity. Soon after arrival you bought them pails, shovels, and sunscreen. They tanned to adulthood. You followed every California craze, from turkey burgers to tofu, you the orthodox cantor's daughter, no wonder your voice held such music.

I never told you Irv called. I wouldn't have added to your guilt. In less than a year he remarried anyway. And you, who wanted the freedom, got lonely. I heard it in the frequency of your Saturday night calls, and their length. There was a certain illogic when you left him, which stung me, resonated with the way my husband, Michael, had just moved out. All those promises, honey on Rosh Hashanah apple slices, promises for a sweet New Year, promises of love, and until-death. I wanted to believe so much in people's words then; innocent and ignorant, a flower child.

Because I was in medicine, I held cause and effect sacred too. That first marital failure of mine destroyed my belief in logic. It's the heart that governs after all. The head, stuffed with reasonable utterances, turns out to be utterly useless. Still, those were first divorces. We could, and did, lay responsibility, like a death wreath, at their door. The cleanest explanation for why was yours, years later. *You never know what goes down in a marriage, unless you sleep between the sheets with them.*

You were at Colette's bedside, later in the week. She was awake, stable, moving her extremities, when you called me mid-morning, hopeful. I told you then Lamar had asked me to marry him.

"You're not learning unless you're failing," you sang. "Go ahead, marry him. Try."

I've been intimidated by change forever. I vacillate, so long a habit, it's a character trait now. My first divorce destabilized me badly, the very word wife made my palms sweat. Naturally my first husband had to leave. I never could have decided, despite the rot.

You were Ms. Impulsive. But that week with Colette, you wanted certainty like never before. I wondered if you were encouraging me to cliff-walk, so we could trade places. I might become bold and you would happily behave predictably.

You were relieved to have Lily and Irv close, but they brought up other issues. "Sometimes with Lily, I don't know," you'd said. "She went and told Colette how I was when we first moved here. Claims she was only a child herself. And I made her make dinner three nights a week, baby-sit. She was eleven, for heaven's sake. I made her set the table. Like I dated so much then. I was always home before midnight. Never went out during the week, unless it was an audition.

"All right, I met a few mistakes. That Romanian gypsy who moved in with us didn't believe I was trying out for plays; threatened to cut me when he caught me rehearsing a script with someone. Okay, the methadone addict, another error. But he worked in a stereo store, made good money. He was an engineer, and Jewish, for God's sake. The worst, the worst though, was that wacko TV exec. A goy. Bipolar. On coke. God we had fun. Filthy rich, very exciting. Well of course he had to be wealthy at the rate he snorted. It didn't matter so much then, money. But now, aging, it's taken on weight, like everything. Face creams, body oils, eye-tucks, hair-color, gym memberships. Our mothers should've warned us."

"Relax Nola, you're beautiful. You'll always be beautiful," I said. "It's my hair that's gone dull as pewter."

You began humming, *Hush little baby* to Colette and I knew you weren't with me any longer. "Doctor's here, gotta go. I'll let you know anything when I do. Thanks so much for listening." You made three kiss sounds into the receiver and said, "Do it. Marry him."

Colette's recovered completely. Our daughters define themselves by autonomy now; act as if they're making adulthood up, fresh. They believe what they declare will come into being, immediately, and will remain until they choose differently. They burn through youth, spin by lovers, heave friends away, tilt at career windmills, and slam too many doors. We should warn them about sheering forces, about how cumulative defeats will mar them, but we're almost wise now, so we stay silent.

I still remember your forty-fifth. You called and said, "I've made a late Jewish New Year's resolution. Can you even do that for Rosh Hashanah? Well never mind, *No more men unless they have deep lines beside their eyes. I have to know they're able to laugh.*"

The night before my surgery, it was past one a.m. when fatigue finally registered. I thought about getting off the phone; I had to be in the hospital by five. But if I hung up, I should go to bed. He'd come out earlier, scowled and sliced at his throat for me to cut it off, then slammed away, the door rattled after him. I clung to your chatter like a fevered child, a voice against the dark.

You went back to Lily again. "Her therapist says *I* want to keep her infantile and dependent, that she must not contact me. Can you believe it? Irv's paying this woman good money. When I get through to Lily, I warn her, she's got to switch, she's not a trained therapist, she's a witch."

There's a long pause then, as if we're each waiting for new shoes.

"I called her last week and said, 'Come home for Rosh Hashanah, Lily. 'I'll make your favorites, overnight cholent, chocolate mint pie. I'll give you the complete recipes this time, I won't leave anything out. This way, you'll always know something sweet and nutritious.'"

My hand cramps with the writing. I hear your voice, joshing me. *Oh, honey, it's too much coffee, too much solitude, birthday jitters.* I hear your laughter, wind through aspen leaves when they're still green, firmly attached. *Five days without presents, no lover, without anyone. The accident's too fresh. You're just spooked, is all. Here, take my hand,* you say, and I hold mine out. The waitress refills my coffee and my hand doesn't dare tremor in this café of strangers.

The sun spiked yellow between clouds as the paramedics surrounded the children, the mother and father, started IVs. They took pulses, clamped monitors, slammed ambulance doors. I palmed my eyes against the glare, escaped to a thin blue rim of mind, away from the smell of blood and molten metal. I rubbed the back of my hand on my forehead then, hard, wiped both palms on my jeans, but the blood stains stuck to my skin. I'd have to stop to wash up, put on a fresh shirt, brush my hair before Taos.

I drove slower after the wreck, heard Lily's voice on the phone. I misheard her at first, thought it was you. Her pitch was a little too high, the voice broken, as though she'd swallowed glass. She said how they found you: slumped over the edge of the tub at your girlfriend's apartment, six a.m. Your nebulizer was still clutched in your hand, breath clamped out by small muscular contractions, your trachea and bronchi in an acute asthmatic attack. You had stayed the night because they were treating your apartment for roaches, again. All those years we knew each other, family dinners, camping trips, later, our pajama parties, I'd never seen an inhaler, never heard a wheeze. Never. Never saw you use those small accessory collarbone muscles to help you breathe.

The entire drive over Raton Pass was a time of bargaining. *I'll be good, I'll never swear again, I swear. I'll mend old wounds, be civil to both my ex's. I'll behave better, I'll be kinder, I'll do anything, just spare our children. Give me time.*

When Lily spoke, I took your postcard from the mantel and pressed it to my abdomen, thickly bandaged and sore as hell. When I hold you now Nola, you're in that scar. It began as a long red welt, thick as a menstrual pad, ruining my belly. After they took the stitches out, it shriveled to a pink pucker, like the butt of a breech newborn. And now, when I touch it, your voice helps me with fear. The way you did when my first husband left. I had no idea how to raise children, balance a checkbook, take the car for repairs, how to be alone. The issues are different now, the fear's constant.

Tell me, you say, *what are you most afraid of?*

Death, I answer.

And how many years do you think you have left? Go inside, think hard, even with Parkinson's. Meditate before you answer, you say.

My fingers slide down the thin midline ribbon of flesh, white, rippled, pouty. Narrow as a scalpel blade. *The average lifespan's twenty years from diagnosis.* I've done my homework after Mother's death. *Ten of them good.*

What did you expect then, immorality? You laugh, with the fine high ring of expensive crystal.

Nola, I'll always miss you.

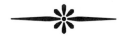

My son Ben was a very active child, inquisitive, a jumping boy. One afternoon when the neighborhood children were playing in our backyard, one raced inside, screaming that Ben had hurt himself, was bleeding. My son stood by the fence, crying and staring at his hand, the blood dripping freely down his arm. I put pressure on the wound, held it high, carried him inside, wedged against my hip, washed it. As soon as it was level with his heart again, the bleeding resumed. The cut gaped, and I felt faint, thinking my boy's lifeblood is running down the drain. I wrapped his hand in gauze, immediately pink, then red, and carried him next door. Stitches poked my brain, but I couldn't unwrap and examine it again. Never mind the myriad of small hands I'd sutured in the ER in Philadelphia. This was my child.

I asked my neighbor to look, tell me if he needed the hospital. Of course he did. She drove, I kept the pressure on. Five stitches. He healed fine.

The Date, The Rape & Dad

The Date

Iris breezed into my life in the mid-'70s from back East, from Jersey. She'd just moved to Denver and her mother, close friend of my ex's aunt, told her to call me, said I was a mensch. "Avoid the nephew," Aunt Enid continued. "The man's tall, very good looking, but he's treated her like a schmuck."

It was a free-wheeling time, lots of left-over hippie hype, love-ins, and relatively safe sex. Transmitted diseases were embarrassing, inconvenient, but a little penicillin fixed you right up. Iris was more adventuresome than I was. I'd been married eleven years, making babies, finishing medical school and pathology training, trying to glue my marriage together a little longer.

Iris tutored me in contemporary dating. The last time I'd gone out, there wasn't even safe birth control. Iris was a sophisticate. She swore the only reason she married during law-school, was because, at twenty-eight, divorcée sounded sexier than single.

After she settled into her new job and apartment, I talked her into a Car Care For Women course at AAA. It was the first night I'd been out in months, but my car was falling apart, my budget tight. AAA tried to make us more paranoid than we already were as single women. Their message was, *a woman driving alone into a service station equals easy money*. The two things I remember thirty years later is if someone's looking under your hood, no matter the weather, or how dressed up you are, get out and stick your head under too. "Do it," they commanded, "even if it looks like wet spaghetti on a wall. Your presence alone will intimidate most attendants."

They showed a knife-ring gizmo, available to sleazy attendants who could, and would, slice your fan belt or radiator hose unless your face were six inches away from theirs. AAA showed tapes of women driving cross-country, stopping for gas off the interstate, ruined by outrageous repairs, a "frayed" alternator hose, or tire replacement. We saw a razor device filmed as it shot out of a shoe like a snake tongue, slashed the tire, slipped back in: a sole switchblade.

It seemed ludicrous for two professional women to spend Tuesday evenings listening to such warnings, but Iris flirted with the red-headed instructor, fabulous buns, and we stuck it out. We had to change our own oil to graduate. That was the second thing I remember, how easily Iris coerced him to use her car as the demo. I never went near that gooey black slime again.

Iris's man-savvy seemed encyclopedic. After I'd known her awhile, I wondered about genetics. She told me about her mother, widowed three times, all men dying in her arms. "In ecstasy," Iris laughed, although the first husband had been her own beloved father. Iris didn't have a reverent bone in her body. Family legend, after the third death, was that her mother needed to "recuperate." Truth was, Iris quit clerking for some important judge, returning home to put her Mom in an asylum for awhile. Afterglow.

Iris had been dating a "gentleman" in Tulsa, flew there every other month. The man was repulsed by menstruation. Before each tryst, she visited her gynecologist, like having her teeth polished, and had a vacuum extraction of her uterine lining, a mini D&C, even if it weren't near her time. She never told me until real trauma hit, and then she got very confessional. On her return from one of those trips though, she called for a prescription for Qwell because she couldn't face her regular doctor. "My pubes look like they're on fire, almost bleeding from scratching. I can see the little white critters scurrying around. Son of a bitch."

In the mid-'70s, the only real safety precaution on a date was to figure out if he were "normal." Parameters for normal were broad. Honesty was deeply embedded in the counter-culture, contrary to current myths about that time. But I was cautious, an uptightness leftover from '50s high school and a little residua of Catholicism. Wine usually mellowed me to almost happening, almost cool. Iris was always ready to rock. I had three small children; I was never spontaneous.

Exactly how to screen for perverts wasn't clear. It wasn't in self-help books. Lucky me though, Iris had rules. If you haven't been introduced, that is, you don't know him from work or through friends, meet him twice in public, before going to his pad. Watch his behavior before the first "time." Carefully. *Never* consider going to your place the first few times. You don't want him to know where you live. And, this was her one imperative: design the first evening early, with a cut-off excuse like, "My baby-sitter has to be home by ten." You can always renegotiate.

Iris's fail-safe option was to go to his place with another couple. Safety in numbers. Drive your own car. Don't get sloshed. Stay alert.

Counter-culture or no, admitting you had children wasn't smart, Iris insisted. Bad form, unnecessary pressure, until you really knew him. I'd already learned that, on a date with a gorgeous Israeli radiologist I'd met at tumor board. Deep-set, pondering eyes, crevices for dimples, and a head of black curly hair that could snag your fingers for hours. Our first date was to see the Rockies, a third-string hockey team new to Denver. Sports wasn't my forte, but this event involved a lot of screaming and beer. And he was sweet, held the car door for me, gave me a single calla lily wrapped in butcher paper, tied with string. We kissed on my porch after, when my son's trike caught his peripheral vision. His tongue was still in my mouth as he pointed with his eyes, questioning what he was seeing. He'd already agreed to a cup of tea and more conversation inside. "What's that?' he asked and my mouth registered cold autumn air, tannin and tin.

I must've looked puzzled. "Ben's trike." I said. But even in dim porchlight, I saw those dimples flatten, jaws clench, his skin pale to ash.

"Ben?"

"My son. Almost four."

"You have a child?" His arms unwrapped and pulled away so quickly, even my sweater didn't save me from the October chill.

"I have three," I said. It was probably self-preserving that I put the key in the door, pushed with one hip, holding the lily, and reached for his hand. But he was already on the sidewalk, backing to his car, mumbling, "I have to meet John early, to run, early rounds too." Inside, I slid to the floor as he pulled away, roaring recklessly down our small inner-city street. I cried for two hours, then reached the kitchen, crushed the lily, and filled a soupbowl with the children's three-flavored ice cream, hoping he'd blow a rod, or at least get ticketed.

I didn't do bars, so Iris went to those alone, weekends. By early November she found George and they were well into their affair by the holidays: a small gold heart, eighteen carat, with a tiny ruby in the center. That's when I met Richard. A hospital Christmas gala at my partner's home. There was a clown, musicians, and wine and pot, as if none of us would be called the next day to read an emergency bone marrow or do a frozen section of a child's tumor. My partner's wife and long-time friend was a volunteer at the art museum. She'd invited the curator, Richard. He was tall, debonair, and blond, with one of those elongate Scandinavian heads whose perfect shape makes you want to hold it in both hands, sheer tactile joy.

A museum director can't be quirky, I thought. And he was very attentive. He wasn't my type; I liked smaller men, craggier, but New Year's was around the corner. He was suave, intelligent in the way that fund-raisers are, and hip. He was fluent in Western history, classical music, contemporary literature, and jet-set gossip. These were areas I'd had little time for, but they were more interesting than the powder pack at A Basin, or the latest

New England Journal prognosis for rhabdomyosarcoma. Especially at Christmas.

I mentioned Richard's name to my partner and he talked to his wife. A month into the New Year, they played matchmaker, had several couples over for an intimate dinner, plus Richard. And me. It was the kind of Saturday supper I used to give when I belonged to someone.

Richard was charming, conversed about an upcoming tapestry exhibit from Belgium from the Middle Ages. The average weaving had taken four years to complete, done by at least three young women, nimble fingers, impeccable eyesight. The design was by a male artist. Later, in front of the fireplace with a brandy, he described his private litho collection, from the turn of the 19th century. His resonant baritone swelled and coated my ears. In retrospect, his words wove a blindfold around all judgment. His vocabulary almost glistened, and I turned and noticed huge, feathery snowflakes behind beveled glass windows.

Early the next week, he called and asked me for dinner at the "in" restaurant. Saturday night. In the code of the time, this meant he was unattached, Iris told me. The restaurant was upscale; I had nothing to wear, but Iris rescued me, loaned her black cocktail dress, which clung to my hips. Wednesday Ben got chicken pox, a mild case. I called to warn Richard, because it can be terrible in adults, sterility, hospitalization-high fevers. He was nonplussed, had had it as a child, was immune. He didn't even mind that I had three small children. It was a new year.

Friday night about eleven Iris called, frantic. She was in the ER, hemorrhaging from her vagina. No pain, but she was terrified. It was too late for me to get a sitter, so she came to my house by cab, sedated, and I put her to bed in my room. She was better in the morning, groggy when she told about George, about the "double date." She'd been sleeping with him for months, they'd planned a Cancun vacation in April, when he told her he wanted to try something a little different. His cousin was in town, had picked up some trampy vixen, and they shared a pizza and two pitchers, then went back to George's. Both couples made out on matched leather couches in the living room, as if it were a competition. TV light soiled the air. Finally, his cousin and date were naked and retreated to his bedroom, where too-thin walls didn't dampen anything. The sounds aroused George; Iris never needed much start-up. They began what had become pattern, but then George stopped, got up and said, just a minute. She was curious, but hot mostly, and thought, oh the French ticklers he's talked about. Or maybe a *menage à* four. But the bedroom door stayed closed. He came back from the bathroom erect, no protection, one hand behind his back. He mounted her quickly, fine with Iris, and she came within minutes. He was still hard, she could feel him when he started playing with her again, using his hand. That was when she felt something sharp, a streak of pain, then hot liquid. She thought maybe she imagined the pain, the hot wet was his, but it continued. She touched herself; he'd rolled off, and brought a finger to her face. Even in the bluish flicker, she recognizes the dark stain. And the salt smell of blood. She looked between her legs and saw she was still bleeding. She grabbed her underpants, stuffed them under her, and yelled.

George had gone back to the bathroom, returned when she hollered. The bedroom door opened. They all helped her dress; everyone was scared. She had a towel beneath her in the back seat as George sped to the ER, dropped her off, vanished. The bleeding didn't stop. She was shaking her head at my kitchen table Saturday morning, the sleeves of my robe hung over her finger tips.

"A sharp slice, like a razor, the ER doctor said. In my vagina. I can't believe this. I thought we were an item. I was really into George. Three stitches, that fucker. The resident said I was lucky, as if he saw this everyday."

I was having trouble incorporating her facts, which sounded like a scare tactic AAA would use. Suddenly, despite the abysmal years toward the end, my marriage didn't seem that bad. I put Richard off a week with some lame excuse about another child getting chicken pox. Iris's mother flew out and stayed with her, but within a month, stitches out, insides mended, Iris was back at the bars. By then I'd had my own adventure.

I met Richard outside the restaurant, drove my own car. I'd painted my toenails tea-rose that afternoon, even shaved my legs, but not my pits, still a feminist, *au natural*. We had delicious veal Marsala, and he selected a full bodied Rhone, mildly fruity, interesting. Then he ordered an expensive Sauterne with bananas foster to share for dessert. I was beyond mellow, and even in those days, when I sometimes drove slightly tipsy, I knew I'd had too much.

We shared a lot of our histories over three hours; he spoke more about tapestries, the way paintings are transformed, how markers were knotted in the warp or maybe it was the weft, to copy the original design. I told him a little of the intensity of frozen sections, about the difficulty diagnosing tumors in kids. I did not say a word about child autopsies. We both skimmed low-lights of wrecked first marriages, examined each other's scars. There was something sensitive in the way he listened, his long head tilted toward his right shoulder, candlelight reflecting from his wire-rimmed glasses. His wife, Doris, had been the first female anchor on a Portland TV station. He respected women with careers, rare for men in the early '70s, especially for men over thirty. He asked, genuinely, about Ben's recovery, and if my third little one had symptoms. A sure-fire shot into this mother's heart. It hadn't hurt that he'd swept my hand to his lips when I first arrived, told me I looked beautiful.

It felt safe to go to his home for coffee, to see his lithos. We would return to the restaurant for my car, after I'd sobered up. He worked with my partner's wife. It never crossed my mind to offer the obvious: the restaurant served espresso. I was horny.

His home was carefully appointed, expensive, authentic antiques. His lithos were extraordinary. He told me how many of each had been made, described the process, the history of the minor artists, whose signatures were still visible. He knew all the gallery owners in New York, and they called if anything in his period was being offered. He visited "the city" every two months, wanted me to accompany him next time. He poured more liqueur and I forgot I was supposed to be on guard. He lit a fire, slipped on the couch beside me, nuzzling and petting until I forgot time.

I'd called the sitter from the restaurant and she checked with her mother; she could stay the night, although I promised to be home by two.

He caressed and warmed my feet in his hands, then slowly slid his fingers up the insides of my legs, thighs, brushed my triangle, pulled his hands away, switched to my face, my hair. It was like he was a sculptor learning my body, his eyes closed, he fingered my forehead, eyebrows and lashes, then lips, which I parted. He only let me nibble a little, worked his fingertips up my cheeks, through my hair, to my scalp. He massaged it in large strong circles. It was a luxury to be touched again. All this idiotic guarding, calculating whether someone was decent enough, employed, not doing hard drugs. He never went near the kitchen for coffee, but I'd forgotten that pretense already.

He unbuttoned my blouse, one hand stroked my neck, his mouth on my breast, his second hand beneath Iris's dress. He whispered my name, said he loved my smell, said anything. He picked me up like I weighed twenty pounds less, carried me to his bedroom, to his California king.

Wouldn't I please try one of his ex-wife's nighties. That rattled me. He must have sensed reluctance, because he lit a candle immediately and began caressing me again. His hand probed me, and before responding, I remembered Iris for a minute. But then I relaxed into his insistence, came quickly. He groaned and nudged a bit longer, but we were both drunk, soon asleep.

Streamers of predawn light slithered between his drapes as his hand rocked my shoulder, heavy, demanding, "Wake up, I've got a surprise."

I was beyond hangover-drunk, almost drugged, tried to focus on his too close face. When my eyes opened fully, they slammed shut immediately, on their own. What I'd seen was a repeat of childhood, only his height and coloring were off. Thick-waisted, long-torsoed, with blond spare chest hairs sprouting through his wife's black lace negligée. Like Dad "playing" in Mom's. Richard stood in a short satin nightie, seams splayed across his hips. The lace hem did not cover his penis, hanging long and pale. I pulled into myself, an automatic, ancient gesture, before I felt his tongue in my ear, "Here, help me, I need your help. I know I can get it up. I've been awake for hours trying. I've never had this kind of trouble with a woman before. It must be your sweetness, you remind me of Doris. When I used to have problems, her satin always helped."

I was suddenly more sober than I'd ever been. I had broken every rule: no car, no one knew exactly where I was, I had gotten totally sloshed, come back to his place voluntarily, had gotten more drunk. Had come, forgodssake. I tired to push him away, but he was six-six, strong, agitated. I whispered I needed the bathroom, slipped out from under him, and stumbled into a closet, filled with negligées, boas, the floor littered with large, open-toed pumps. He'd left that light on, so the long cashmere robe on the mannequin at the back of the closet, whose face looked identical to a photo of his wife on the mantle, made me shiver. I flicked the light off, grabbed the nearest next doorknob, and exited.

There was no switch in the hall for light into the living room, but I smelled the smoke from our fire, found the guest bath, peed, and squeezed my head between my hands, hoping for a plan. I let the water run, tiptoed around the corner, grope-found the phone, dialed O. I was about to speak, it had to be softly, but louder than my heart, when his hand ripped the phone out of mine, and in one swift maneuver, he yanked the cord out of the wall, slammed his hand against my head, and threw the phone across the room. I slid down the wall, was still cowering, when he scooped me up again, carried me back to bed. He was full now, insisted I give him head. I did, until my jaw felt like it was going to lock. Finally, he came. Now the sun was up, the curtains were tangerine, and he immediately fell asleep. The only sound was from the bathroom where the water continued to run down the drain. I untangled myself from his hold, pulled on my skirt and blouse, grabbed my purse, shoes and coat, and left. I walked two miles home, no underwear, no sweater, never felt the late January frost.

I only ever told Iris.

The Rape

I was astonished that my taste for Bordeaux vanished that night. I still recall the exact scent of Richard, years later. Thick alcohol and the once erotic, now tainted, mix of musk and unwashed woodsy mushrooms. One night, one small part of one night, had changed desire forever.

About a year after Richard, I called Iris, ready to rejoin the world. Maybe we could catch a foreign film at Denver University Saturday night. Iris picked me up, and afterward we had a drink at Racine's. We were both considering going on the wagon, soon. Iris dropped me off, drove the sitter home. It was around eleven when I checked the children, all asleep, including the giggly blonde Ariel had as a guest. The girls arms lay tangled carelessly in each other's hair.

I took a long bath, reheard Iris's tales of her latest hottie; her talk rekindled something I thought extinct. I willed myself back to the spectacular green of the Irish countryside in the film, a color bleached from Denver by August, gone until spring. I went to bed around midnight, read three pages, turned off the light.

It was an event like a childhood bee sting, unexpected, undeserved, full of terror. A shock produced by a tiny insect so that afterward, I was temporarily paralyzed, could only retrieve strobed bits. Remembering, trying to remember, had the effect of visual flicker, patches of sun splintering unevenly through trees on certain roads late afternoons, a scratch at the brain, close to convulsion.

That first week following the rape, a word I never spoke out loud, was emotionally flat. But later, with the therapist pounding for a reaction, and her bills mounting, the stone in my abdomen seemed a little lighter. After a month, I started to return. It wasn't voluntary, more like some part of me thought, *enough*. I worried if I dove all the way back, I'd unglue. I wondered how incest victims continued, where they found the will to force themselves to breathe.

I laughed at my first solution later, ridiculous, a year of high necked blouses, long sleeves, even in the heat of summer, and sweltering, floor-length skirts. As if covering flesh could ward off evil. A passionless year, as though punishing my body would atone for the sin. Only, it wasn't my sin.

The rape had, in a split second, well, several slow-motion minutes, shut down pacifism. I even shopped for a handgun before Iris reminded me of the statistics of firearms at home. And my three small, inquisitive children. I snapped back then, but for the better part of that year, I believed capital punishment was appropriate for certain crimes.

Four years later, at a dinner party with liberal colleagues, I made a mini-oration, "I think castration's eminently reasonable. Rape's a very, very violent crime. Serial rapists, pedophiles, cut their nuts off," I raised my half-empty glass of Chardonnay. "Stop testosterone if you intend to release those fuckers."

The hostess tried to shift the discussion to Denver's air pollution, but I would not be silenced. "Talk-therapy does just so much. Alone, it's like heaving a bag of marshmallows on a bonfire." I finished the wine, which tasted sour. For much of the late-'70s, I sounded mainstream, honestly believed violence was a solution.

I spoke the full details only once, told the policewoman that night, while waiting for the doctor in the ER. I'd insisted another policeman stay at my home while I went to the hospital, in case, like he'd threatened, he returned.

I offered money first, hoping it was robbery. Then I feigned an epileptic seizure, a great, detailed job, frothed at the mouth, writhed, stiffened, but the jerky movements hadn't deflected him. In fact, they seemed to irritate him. That was when he rammed the metal rod against my ear, so hard, pain shot through my head, and I wept, silently. It was then I knew she had little choice. So what if he lied, if only half his statements were true? He had the gun. His truth became hers, and he became, for a stopped moment, her world.

In the ER I regained enough of myself to insist the doctor test for gonorrhea and syphilis. Had it been a decade later, I'd have included AIDS. I refused to drink or swallow the water the policewoman offered until oral cultures were obtained, his residual semen a pearl paste over back teeth, secluded in the recesses of my tonsils.

I startled awake when he cracked the door open. A little after one a.m. on the alarm clock. Time exploded during the act, an endless, immediate physicality, until she ascended to a ceiling corner where she stayed as he entered. Her thoughts sped through every option, metal against her skull erased emotion. She was as impotent as all that useless data in rape-prevention pamphlets.

I had always parked beneath street lamps; always insisted someone escort me to my car after dark, leaving the hospital; had always, always, locked car doors. And if alone, before I started the engine, I'd never shut my door completely until I'd felt the backseat, ready to jump out at first contact.

I'd attended medical school in Philly, in the ghetto, during the race riots of the '60s. I knew the ways to behave in public, if an assailant had a weapon: jagged running into a street, an improbable target. I knew that escape during the early part of an incident is the best chance of survival you'll ever have. To scream, to run toward a crowd, to yell *Fire*, not *Rape*. I knew the collapse of all defenses at the end of the booklet: if caught and armed, that is, if he is armed and you are caught, to submit. And if you are armed, to shoot, to kill.

I remember details as if they were branded. The metallic ice of his hands against the warm flesh of her inner thighs. The rough, barbed-wire bristle of that exploration. His finger tips wore jagged calluses, a manual laborer. But his palms were covered in wool. Even at the time, she knew that was bizarre. She thought of golf gloves, which covered the palm in suede, left the fingers free; but golfer fingers would be white-collar protected, soft appendages. His were coarse.

Two years later on a cross country ski trip, I saw them. In a shop where the manager was pushing the new, all-temperature wax, I froze in front of a stack of huge gray gloves. There they were: spiky country wool, mitten ends that peeled back, to cover, or expose, finger tips. Quirky equipment for an arduous sport, before it became techno-competitive.

Too often she could still close her eyes and see his silhouette against the mandala above the dresser. She threw out the sheets and nightie immediately. Eventually, repainted the room, periwinkle, even the ceiling. She re-arranged the furniture. She'd estimated him at five-ten, because his shoulders intersected the macramé circle there. She'd used a measuring-tape to check. That reference point, his shadow-image, kept her focused, centered her in the way a mantra might have, had she been calm enough to recite one.

His dark outline scared her, forced her not to faint, not to laugh hysterically, not to scream. She had only seen his figure for a few seconds, before he demanded she shut her eyes, pull her pillowcase over her head. "Or I'll blow your head off. Now just do as I say and you won't get hurt. And I won't do those four young ones, either. If you holler and wake them, I'll shoot the whole bunch of you."

I can no longer comfortably go to a bar where the floor-boards stink of soaked whiskey. Male armpit odor, once adored, smells like burned flesh in my nose. When I finally began to date, if there was any hint of liquor, even faint mouthwash on the man's breath, I was pounded to nausea, identical to first trimester.

For the first six months, I thought I would recognize that voice forever. It was seared in my ear, right next to the metal. I answered the phone hesitantly and actually shivered if the voice were male, a baritone. I paused, held my breath, and waited for the graveled impediment. Not a stutter exactly, just a suggestion of difficulty with large, polysyllabic words. He never called.

I was edgy around strangers, and that persisted, years after therapy.

Near dusk that first week, before I bought the Rott-
weiler and had grills welded on the basement windows,
where the police had found large footprints and broken
glass, I wondered if this were some dark, karmic joke, inverted because I had so rejected my Republican family-of-
origin. I wondered if I were being punished for trying the
precepts of Gandhi's satyagraha in America; maybe they
didn't translate across cultures. Perhaps I'd weakened my
natural survival instinct with blind devotion to peace.

I rotated back through that night again and again, trying to assess if she'd genuinely believed, as he threatened,
that he would "do" her children. I rubbed my forehead
with the back of my hand so often, it started to break
out. I tried to erase the memory, postpone the migraine.
Most nights I made supper, for the children at least. The
days were easier, my work was, of necessity, intense and
absorbing. Dressing and undressing the children were
still tactile pleasures. Touching my own body, a different
thing entirely.

The holidays were a challenge that year. I did the eight
nights of lights and gifts for the children, but New Year's
Eve hung ugly and naked. Michael had the children that
week. Iris invited me to a "hair do" party, hired a stylist
and colorist, asked a barber-friend too. I thought it was
going to be a coed Tupperware type evening, wigs, new
styles to fight the January blahs. I was underdressed in a
turtleneck and jeans, wore my hair down in a prim silver
barrette, hoped I'd be chosen for the experiment, dyed
or curled, I was ready for change. The guests arrived in
flowing gowns and tuxes. When Iris came downstairs, she
was stunning in a magenta sari. Iris's hair, well words
didn't, couldn't, it was like a resurrection: her skull was
parceled into separate patches, each colored and styled
differently. There was a periwinkle wave over her right
ear, tiny cornrows with blue beads in the back, a large
purple pompadour above her widow's peak, a maroon
Afro haloed her left ear, and salmon pin-curls exposed
scalp on the crown. The nape of her neck was edged by
short-cropped, green hair, like a lawn in which a buzz

cut maze was carved, so compelling that all night male fingers followed its furrows, a few strayed lower. Each time Iris responded with a shudder and a growl.

I left early, feeling dowdy, but enchanted by Iris's unwavering efforts, her willingness to return to the playing-field, no matter. The next morning I awoke nettled by a nubbin of envy, the first blush of health. It wasn't much later, early February, that I agreed to a night out, just the two of us, to a small blues bar off Market and 20th.

Two weeks after it happened, I made my second call to the police, spoke with a friend of a friend who came to my home and made safety recommendations: deadbolts, floodlights, bars on the basement windows, and a dog, a big dog. He was an older detective who agreed to search the police files thoroughly, to check if there were an MO for a similar perp, the half-exposed hands, the pillowcase, the gun. I knew the average rapist didn't pack, or have the temerity to enter a private home. I'd never heard of a rapist so repulsed by menstruation that he'd switch gears, insist on fellatio. Such imagination, the pillowcase, peeled up enough so just her mouth was exposed. The first real laugh I had that first month was when Iris lamented, "If only *my* ex had been that perverse, I'd still be happily married."

When I let myself think about it, he'd actually been macho, trusting himself inside her mouth. She had sharp incisors. Wasn't there a real possibility that terror or rage or nervousness might misfire, cause her to bite the damned thing off? Ballsy of him, really.

And years later, after my second divorce, when my children are grown and I've filled their rooms with a large weaver's loom, oily wool in natural hues, I permit myself an occasional passionless liaison, in search of a good man. After each affair, I need a light in the dark again.

Slowly, my yearning for revenge reversed, at a glacial pace, and I slid back to non-violence. My steps are bouncier; I wear clothes with a lilt of sensuality, and find myself out alone, late. True, I whistle into the tunnel of darkness, but I'm out.

& Dad

Sometimes the way to survive is to compartmentalize. You put certain information in a little box, tie a blue ribbon around it, if joyful, go on. The birth moment of each child; early marriage months, first marriage; the spectacular shades, violet, pearl gray, peach, bone-white that spin the façade of the Taj, touring northern India; the first sunrise you and your second husband witness, a beach in Kauai; the sky, dark with bald eagles near Haynes, a birding extravaganza after your first divorce; your daughter, Tori's with you, she's eight. There was the way your mother apologized once, actually said she was sorry, for failures during your youth. You are thirty-eight at the time, it's a year after your first divorce, the evening before your tubal. You are bathing. Your mother sits on the throne, lid down, offers to soap your back, admits she didn't protect you from your father. She hadn't known any better, had done the best she could. Inadequate to your close friends, like Iris, who know some of your childhood stains. But it gives you the space to repair three years from your early thirties, fresh out of Payne Whitney, when you refused to speak with your folks at all, a chance to "make up" with Mom, before her mind becomes wispy, itinerant, finally vanishes.

And yes, your father had always been odd, less like other blue-collar dads in the neighborhood, whom you silently admired, some nights even wished were yours. Those dads worked shipyards and oil refinery jobs in Elizabeth and Newark, rough-housed their kids, swatted them for misbehaving, hollered and all, but they also picnicked with them in the park, went to the shore summer weekends, and hugged them hard at night. You saw it. They screamed encouragement at track meets or softball games and were awed by good grades.

Your household didn't acknowledge physical achievements. Your father was a teacher, had asthma so bad that any effort not applied to breathing or making a living was considered frivolous. Your parents expected grades of one hundred percent. You defended every missed point, had to. There were a few memories of drama, the ambulances with oxygen for Dad's attacks, the tip-toeing around him for weeks afterward. Your relief going to school then, where the air wasn't thick with wheezing, and medicine.

There were tortured battles between your parents when your father wasn't sick. Your mother would draw the curtains in the daytime, homesick herself, head between her hands, nails bitten to bleeding cuticles, face ribboned with tears, swollen. Not bruised physically, mind you, as your own face sometimes was, but distorted by great disappointment. Your father would grow more sullen, slam doors, slam his briefcase of unmarked papers, slam you if you drew too near. And because the apartment was tiny and crowded, all corners cluttered by layers of books and African violets on wobbly stands, sometimes his whacks knocked you down, shoved you into things. *You* broke containers, spilled soil and furry leaves and tiny purple flowers all over the floor. Your mess further infuriated him, sometimes to the point of a belt-beating.

Those episodes spiraled like a rattler coiling, so you would choose to lose count, relax into it, breathe, strike, breathe, pain, breathe, don't scream, until you willed yourself small, then grown-up, a tiny speck of an old maid. Sometimes your mother came during the rhythmic thwaps, mumbled an appeal that stopped him. But the older you grew, the more often you had to endure the full fury, until he was frothing, until he reversed the belt so the buckled-end bit your flesh, your bottom crimsoned before he'd stop. Sometimes you wondered if you'd survive. But if you kept those beatings in small packages, never thought about them afterward, for days or months even, you could enjoy the taste of milk and fig newtons at school.

The rest of the memories lay buried. In sealed envelopes you hope, which you never intend to open. Even though you'll spend years in therapy, you never reach farther back than seven, maybe six once, toward your sister's birth, your baby brother's birth and death, a few times to pre-Daddy, to when you lived in the purring of your grandparent's home, songs on their Victrola, great-granny beside you at night, snoring in her bed in that Brooklyn brownstone. There, you were "cutie," taken to Prospect

Park Zoo every Sunday by your grandfather, you have the pictures to prove you were coddled and worshipped. You stay in therapy while you raise your children, the cost in terms of dollars, time or pain irrelevant, because you know you hold the same tantrums Dad exhibited, feel them lurch toward the surface periodically. Your frustrations and fatigue with exceedingly long work weeks, the grind of single-parenting, stretch you too often toward that unmanageable rage. You are afraid of yourself, and what you carry.

Now you're at your father's bedside in Miami Baptist Hospital. He's in intensive care, and you've flown down from Detroit, standby, first flight out. His hip fractured, which his home-aide eventually admitted happened when she stepped onto the patio for a smoke. First story was that he slid under the table while he and his lady-friend ate sandwiches. With further pressing, it turned into a sort of sordid hanky-panky, the paramedics reported him wedged beneath the table, tangled in the lady's underwear. You don't see any reason to explore details further. He isn't doing well. The hip looked hideous, you studied the pre and post op films yourself. The orthopedist's original estimate of "an hour, max" stretches to four and a half. You know what a bad long-term prognosis that is.

But you're determined to see this through. No matter how many nurses you disturb, how many specialists you hound, you insist his lungs and heart and brain are cared for, aggressively. You pray the wound heals rapidly, doesn't get infected. Your sister cannot get back, cannot be reached most days. It would be unthinkable if she could not say her final goodbye.

It's three years since you've been to Miami, your mother's antique face imprinted one last time before burial. You witnessed your father's military back bend slightly then. You've renewed your girlhood friendship with your sister, who's done all the caring for your ailing parents, she, the good daughter. And now your sister and her husband (first and only) have flown to the Far East, tour Japan, Thailand, China, a well-deserved Asian vacation. You are the designated keeper of your father's well-being for the month. You cannot make this decision alone. How did your sister manage all these years?

You're on call at your own hospital when you receive the surgeon's message, trade the beeper to your partner. The surgeon refused to take the eighty-three-year-old to the OR unless a member of the immediate family were present.

You are a few years past the bad body-flashbacks of early childhood. These struck during the dying days of your last marriage, as it bled brutal and scary enough, so even you no longer dared go on the yacht alone with him.

Fear's an interesting whip, careens your body and mind between what is now: you, a mature woman, armed with resources and intelligence and that familiar immobilizing childhood, that long spread of helplessness. During that final chapter of your last love, you found yourself at an age you didn't want to be, you were young again, you didn't really know how young, but there you were, defenseless, and with part of you, down there, ripping. You feel your bottom tear, hear muffled screams, smell your father's adenoidal breath hot against your neck. At first you were certain this was your mind's perverted way of dealing with another failed relationship, your mind distancing you from this stupid same-error: divorce again. You were having false memories. Your soon-to-be-ex, a Mormon, agreed. He'd met your parents, admitted your dad was a strange duck, but hadn't that same dad taken you on hikes in the woods, you'd told him those stories. And when you think about it, Dad was the one who taught you how to hold a snake and not blink as it slithered cool and sleek through your fingers. He showed you how to put cotton and twigs in a shoebox and use an eyedropper to feed a porridge of bread and milk to a fledgling bird. Hadn't he sworn he loved you? Always, like each of your husbands.

Even your sister, who was one of the first, beside Iris, to encourage you to go back into therapy when you began getting body signals, your sister, who spent ten years as a social worker for battered women and children, insisted that with your continuous putrid selection of men, you must have been incested. Your behavior was textbook classic. Your sister pushed and nudged, even suggested hypnotherapy. But your sister wanted the recall name to be grandfather, and that's not what was in the envelope.

The early part of the week rotates around failing organs, fluid to keep his asthma in check, treatment for his overloaded heart, and once that's addressed, there's renal shutdown, prostate trouble, rounds and rounds of specialists with their entourages and drips and studies. Dad's kept pain free, incoherent a few hours on Monday. The rest of the week he's completely alert, has the staff laughing. He knows who you are and thanks you by name for chipped ice. You read him the comics, fetch his lady friend, spend too much time in the hospital. You keep late night vigils with him until Friday, when you really need to get out for awhile. So after his dinner, you tell him the good news, the doctors think he's improved enough to be moved to a post-op surgical floor tomorrow. You lean over to kiss his cheek you shaved yourself that morning, and say, "Dad, you know I remember everything you ever did to me. And Dad, that was a long time ago. I forgive you. We can start a new relationship now, let's start over."

You rehearsed this last night, are mostly relieved it's been said. A part of you is repelled by this goody two shoes behavior. Another part thinks that if his organs collapse, at least you'll have eased his passing. And behaved magnanimously, maybe there's a reward for that. No, you know better.

He nods his head sadly, as if you could start again, says, "Sure honey, now go get yourself something to eat. See you in the morning."

You've been put off by the high regard the staff has for him, the great gent. All his regular physicians like him, but three weeks isn't forever; you'll manage. You're annoyed by the way he introduces you these last two days. When asked who this is, he says, "Oh, this is my elder daughter, Miss Drink Your Liquid, Miss Pain in the Ass." Everyone thinks he's cute. You try to correct him once, but it's as futile as when you were ten. Or five.

Back in your motel that night, you realize it's nearing March eighth, the problematic anniversary date. It's twenty plus years after the rape, and still it's there. A certain collision of sensations inevitably send you back. If you lay in the dark, in a bed with the door immediately to your left, you can't get your eyes to stay closed. In the night, especially around one a.m., if you're alone and there's the slightest noise, the hint of a step outside the door, you sit bolt upright and remain alert for hours. If you go out with someone new and he has firm, thick fingered hands, you become jumpy. If a man, even a close, long-term friend, runs work-roughened fingers over your skin, it could be a place as non-intimate as your elbow, you shudder. You pour yourself a half glass of scotch, put the TV on loud, order room service, and finally fall asleep around three.

When you awake Saturday, later than you'd intended, you shower quickly but by the time you get to the hospital, you're damp from hurrying, and your father's bed is empty. For a full minute you panic, stomach queasy, and then remember he's been transferred. It takes an hour to round up the nurses, gather his belongings, get directions to the other building, wait for him to be wheeled back from x-ray. He looks particularly happy to see you, his eyes sparkle, which you take as the beginning of something new. You ask if he's eaten breakfast yet, and when he says no, he missed it, you take his order and buy what he wants at the cafeteria. Then you sit on the edge of his bed and offer him banana and sliced oranges. His hand darts out so suddenly you never see it. He grasps your left hand and brings it to him, beneath the flimsy gown and roars, "Do me," yanking the hand up and down. It's so fast, and your arthritis is so bad that it takes you a full series of "No, Daddy, no. No more, you can't do this anymore," before you disentangle your hand and pull back from the bed, now splattered with fruit. He has that air of being right you remember from childhood, the I'm-important-and-you're-toilet-paper façade. You're shaking like you have the DTs when you notice he's reaching to you again, toward your chest this time, a palsied, pill-rolling movement of his left hand. You've worn the filmy cut-velvet vest over your T-shirt today, a little more dressed up for the weekend, for the new beginning. And when you speak, you choose the words very carefully. "You know, when I said I forgave you yesterday, I didn't mean it was okay, what you'd done to me. It was terrible, an abomination. It's just that I meant it was over. And it is over, Dad. Dad, do you hear me, Dad?'

His face stiffens into satisfaction, and then cracks into an almost smug grin as he again stretches close, brushing your vest, clasping.

"What are you doing now?" You hear a hint of hysteria at the end of your question. Maybe he's having a small stroke; he's not making eye contact, not really. Maybe the new room disorients him. Maybe he's more medicated than you think; maybe you look too much like your mother, maybe he's just mixed up. "Dad, do you know who I am?"

"Of course, you're my daughter, you're mine. And what I'm doing is taking that damned shirt away from your breast. I need it."

You leave for Detroit the next day. Beside seeing your therapist, the one person you want is Iris. You need her acerbic wit. You and she managed a few meetings over the years, occasional phone calls, but after she moved, then you moved, it's been difficult. Still, in times of deep stress, it's Iris's cockeyed humor you crave, her irreverence.

Iris had been on the phone the first anniversary of the gun-rape, when you saw fragments of that night re-spool across your kitchen, light spilling from the hall around his shoulders, the smooth cotton pillowcase pressing your nostrils closed, the work of keeping your mouth open so long, the way he had no scrotal hair, the sour, almost vomit smell of him. It was Iris who heard your voice grow shrill, who had the intelligence to ask what was happening, to keep you talking and grounded through the worst of it, who had then come over and spent the night.

Once every few years your mind returns to slick, hairless genitalia, to the absent pubic tangle. The almost-bald scrotum of the rapist blends to the gravid bag of the art director, loose below the black lace hem of the too-tight teddy. And to your father's shriveled, corrugated sac at the margin of his hospital gown, with its countless purple flowers fluttering across the fabric.

Originally you thought, she believed, that feature of sparse hair so particular she'd consulted a colleague in forensic pathology, to check if genital hairlessness was as unique as she suspected, a final clue. But the trail was cold. And then I think, what could I have learned anyway? Nothing about why.

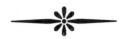

Denver General's ER was one of the worst Saturday night assignments of my internship. A young teenage girl was in the holding cell, and I was supposed to examine her for pneumonia. Before the cell opened, she was cuffed, and her ankles shackled. The guard let me enter her cage. She stood still in her orange jumpsuit, coughed often, as I moved my stethoscope over her chest. She was extremely controlled, did whatever I asked. Deep breath, hold, cough, please. Her eyes stayed on her feet, as if they held an escape plan. She could not have been more than thirteen. I asked her to cough up whatever she could into the specimen cup, capped it for the lab. It was bloody, TB a real possibility. The guard relocked her in, released her hands. She curled eight fingers around the bars, pulled her face close. I leaned in to hear, she could have been my young cousin, a daughter, years from now; so what, she made one stupid mistake. From deep in her chest she lobbed a wad of yellow and red phlegm in my face. She was TB positive. My tine tuberculin test never converted.

ASHES, ASHES

What if time isn't linear, doesn't progress past, present, future. What if time's a construct, invented to thwart terror? What if the entire idea, the nit-picking instruments of measuring, clocks, sand passing through wasp-waist glass, cuckoos, watches, atomic deterioration even, are simply add-ons, so that we humans remain organized, orderly, distracted from the other possibility: that life is simply infinite, simultaneous chaos. Let's say for now that's too hard to think about; let's speak instead of love.

I knew Judson would be disoriented when he stepped off the elevator, so I left the door ajar. Norah Jones' velvet voice filled the third floor hall. *You'll be on my mind forever* ricocheted through the doorjamb, and at his knock, I swallowed my mouthwash. I'd practiced a sultry "hello" all afternoon, but something molecular occurred; an atomic rearrangement sped up my spine when we shook hands. It was central, breath-stealing, left me mute. He's a surfing "bud" of my son, only closer to my age. They met in California a few years back, at the seashore, camping. He goes there with his children, every vacation. Everyone surfs. They drive eighteen plus hours from Colorado, have for twenty years. No place like the ocean. Both he and my son believed no other Coloradan could be that devoted, love curls that much. They were startled to see familiar license plates in the campsite, connected, cooked meals together.

He's friendly with my dog before he shepherds me to his car, a suburban van. He holds my door open. Dinner's in

Evergreen; Denver's city lights are a romantic backdrop, but it could be a cave, we're so lost in each other. It's only when the cleanup crew sweeps around our feet, we notice the restaurant's empty.

He drives me home and we talk and listen until two a.m., then walk the dog. Twelve years smartly single, I have standards. My rules are sequential, like a chemistry experiment. But he draws me in his arms, and I'm going to fail: it's organic chem, junior year. The kiss lasts half an hour before he says, "Either take me upstairs or send me home."

I climb the three flights with the dog, humming *Dayanu*, the Hebrew song my first husband sang at Passover, Rosh Hashanah, any excuse to break out his guitar. *Dayanu, it's enough,* and it is enough, firecracker kisses, full body embrace, conversation of double entendres. Even if tonight is it, I'm resurrectable, Hallelujah. *Dayanu.*

My love of Alice is different, utterly. Closer to what enthusiastic Christians mean with their fish symbols, agape. Though we've been suspected.

Not a medicine dropper's truth in that. We used to get a room together at medical conventions; we're both pediatric pathologists, have known each other since the mid-'70s. We met in Breckenridge, Colorado. My department hosted that interim meeting, the pathology group so small and intimate then, they called themselves a club. Alice is one of two, maybe three people in the universe, that can complete my thoughts with my exact vocabulary and syntax.

Occasionally, we vacation together. Our last big tour was northern India, the mid-'90s, after the International Pediatric Pathology Society met in Delhi. Alice was seeking spiritual simplicity, insulation against aging, like the Sadhus coat their bodies in ash. She wants a second skin of mysticism, a union with God ahead of time, so when death comes, the transition will be tolerable. I went to understand the juncture of sex and death and spirituality that writhes through Hindu sculpture. The West separates these functions antiseptically, but there's a sinuous elation, a twining of creation, destruction, abundance and ecstasy that lives in the stone carvings, particularly those at Khajuraho.

We walked around the lake that Colorado autumn, 1976, gold aspen leaves shimmered in the wind, scrub oak crimson, everything exploding color just before hibernation. The night sky fluttered stars, the way it did when Judson and I left the restaurant. City lights blinked through his windshield, a blanket of homes where people held steady Saturday, lazy in front of the TV, doing supper dishes, reading books after their children were bedded. But we were newborns, stimulated by light, touch-starved.

He and I wanted to feel safe physically, so we did what grownups do, what strangers in dark places do, we talked. The wall of words wormed us closer, like a bunting. In my livingroom we sat apart though, he on the couch, me in my rocker, the one I nursed my children in. I stroked the burnished wooden arms, solid memories.

Downstairs, all safety checks, his HIV status, how many recent sex partners, no physicality till the third date, dismantled. Safe, my body screamed, safe? You've been safe twelve years, dead safe.

I opened my eyes to his face, a close blur, touched his cheek, soft as my ring-shawl from India, that swath of cashmere woven tightly enough to slip through a wedding band. He pocketed his glasses, his hands learned my body, so long without touch, it flamed.

Before Delhi, Alice and I had gone to Ahmedabad, to "center" ourselves at Gandhi's ashram. It was where he spent his adult life, where the salt march had incubated. The city's an international hub of textiles; it was also the epicenter of plague outbreaks, the most recent the year before our trip. The disease erupted and spread as if this were the 12th century. The rat population tripled in four months. Everything's sacred in Gujarat; rodents could not be killed, not even sterilized. Contagion spread across the country, paralyzed New Delhi. Our conference was scheduled for that year, canceled the very last minute, travel quarantines. I'd gotten to JFK when CNN said no planes were permitted in or out of Delhi. I retrieved my bag to return home. It was new luggage, a multi-tiered backpack contraption. I zipped the daypack on, hefted the system on my back, and stepped on the escalator. As

I got off I floated, slow-motion backward, my feet and arms aimed at the ceiling, I teetered on the pack, my skirt over my head: total exposure. Passengers gaped, someone threw a quarter. It took a full minute to pull my arms out of the straps and stand up again. The next year I used a soft sided suitcase, a separate backpack.

I got a reprieve with Judson, too. I spent an anxious Sunday waiting for his call, which finally came. We talked and laughed for over an hour, an unspoken yearning in his voice. Heaven knows what was in mine, relief probably. A new date was set, for a decadent dessert. We'd been so engrossed that first meal, we'd forgotten. My daughter was arriving mid-week, staying with me. There'd be no hanky-panky.

Monday he called midmorning from the bank, after work, again at bedtime. Tuesday he called again late morning, and that became our habit, the hour around noon filled with his voice, his concerns, his life. Then an evening allotment, like a drug, bid, twice a day.

Wednesday evening we went to a loud family restaurant, but the noise and lights receded as we fell into conversation, politics, music, literature, nibbled at appetizers to get to the spooning ceremony. We placed mouthfuls of double-fudge sundae into open, opposite lips. He spoke of ex-wives. I recited the short version of my marriages. We commiserated. We whispered of the saving present of children. His were a decade younger than mine, well, he was younger too. He had two in college, one in high school. He was relieved because that fall his youngest would spend half-time with his mother.

Judson was planning his first solo vacation in twenty-one years, to California, to surf. Four weeks in the future. I nodded, remembered my float trip the summer after my first divorce. My children were with me twenty-four-seven, very young. Michael was to have them for five days. There were twelve other people on the rafts, but I remember being alone on the river for three days. Quiet, freedom, the absence of small needful hands.

As we talked, I heard Alice's warning. *Be circumspect with personal information. Be careful, see what happens over time.*

I did give him a thumb-nail version of my career, how I'd left pathology recently because of arthritis, how I missed looking at slides, and teaching. How lucky I was to still be alive, doing something I love, writing. Judson was the first man I dated since I cut back, then quit medicine, who didn't try to coax me back to my "profession," to my senses, to a financially stable career.

Alice also said, *You don't have to tell him your age, you know. And don't tell a new man about your mental history.*

Judson's first wife had been diagnosed a multiple, then a schizophrenic, later narcissistic personality disorder, by a panoply of psychiatrists. He had little faith in that discipline. He told me how it had been "their problem," her disease, like a foreign object. They'd battled together against it until one day, she ran off. One of her personas left the marriage, abandoned their children, took a lover. She returned a year later, wanted back in, but he and the marriage didn't recover. He reached across the table then, touched my cheek, watched me as he said, "Women find me too intense. They get frightened, split."

"You don't see me running, do you?" I said, placing my napkin to my lips, eyes locked on his. He was a lawyer at a bank; numbers intrigued him. He kept questioning my children's ages, how long I'd been in medical training, practice, adding things up. I finally blurted out my age. "While I'm at it," I said, "you should know I was diagnosed paranoid schiz when I was thirty. Locked up for months."

"Like I said," he smiled, "I don't truck much with shrinks."

In the parking lot we clung to each other like orangutans, kissing, petting, heavy as the moon. Our bodies took charge until the headlights of a security car startled us apart. We laughed and slid into his van, the bucket seats awkward for mature bodies. We continued to try to smudge together until, finally, it was midnight, and we broke our embrace, panting.

Later that night, waiting for my daughter, a slit opened in my mind, like separating venetian blinds, and I grew frightened. About the speed of life rekindled, this super hot nova of exploding intimacy. I had discarded every go slow mantra I'd calculated into my life.

In Ahmedabad, a full moon lit the night Alice and I arrived. Jet lagged, we watched women sing and dance around bonfires, accompanied by rhythmic drumming. Goddess celebrations in our courtyard and down by the river. The moist air carried drum vibrations straight to our bellies.

On the plane from Delhi to Ahmedabad, Alice and I were separated. My seatmate said she'd been raised in Gandhi's Ashram, knew the Mahatma.

"Every rule was enforced," she said, in sing-song British. "Everyone had to be in the dining hall before the last bell, or they didn't eat. Everyone had tasks, even the children. Every minute was accounted for, no idleness.

"Prayers and cleaning, cooking, and more prayers. We had to do all sorts of things. There were no servants." She shook her head, "It taught me a person can get used to anything." She gazed out the window at a long brown line of river. "Of course the Mahatma never cleaned. He came to the dining hall anytime, day or night. Always chose the best fruit, the best vegetables."

Alice and I had studied meditation under a disciple of Gandhi's, Eknath Easwaran, whose writings and translations from Sanskrit were sublime, but whose proscriptions were rigid. Detailed daily discipline, Alice starred. It wasn't that I wasn't willing, but a child would get sick or I'd have three weeks of back-to-back surgical-call or my honey would break up with me again, and I'd need to do relationship triage. Too many nights I piled the children into the car in pajamas at three a.m., so I could freeze the distal end of a bowel resection, tell the surgeon where to pull the ostomy through. Later, there were entire weeks when gathering my teens for supper was an achievement. Meditation I dabbled at, inconsistently.

Both Alice and I toured the Mahatma's ashram in awe. His room was set apart in the back of the compound, just where my seatmate said it stood. A whitewashed adobe building. The door was barred, but the gatekeeper opened the padlock because we had come so far, because we were physicians. We took off our sandals, entered the low-ceilinged room. His sleeping palette, covered in simple homespun, faced a bank of windows overlooking the Sabarmati River. For twenty years this was his home. His spinning wheel and walking staff stood in a corner, and a tiny, angled lap desk on stub legs held an ink bottle, an old nib pen, and ancient yellowed paper. There was a minute replica of the monkey statue, paws over eyes, ears, mouth. No evil.

The second day in Ahmedabad we took a motor rickshaw to a textile museum. Alice is a lifelong knitter and tapestry enthusiast. Peacocks strutted through quiet green gardens, a relief from the streets crammed with buses, trucks and taxis, jockeying camels, elephants, and thin men on motorcycles, thinner ones on bikes. Dust and dung was everywhere. Inside, three stories of delicate, fabulous fabric was folded behind glass. The panels hung on metal spindles, which opened like pages of a book. There was air conditioning, subtle lighting, and a restricted number of visitors. Two guards were actually awake, prowled the cool marble corridors. Marco Polo's cape was glassed in the last room, a magnificent ivory satin, covered with white silk embroidery, twenty square feet. The stitches were so fine, only girls of five or six could have made them.

Outside, sweat, thick curry, and decaying marigolds flavored the air. Young men held each other's hands as they walked by rainbows of cotton on stall shelves. Delicate women in tribal dress wore cheap bangles on fleshless forearms. Everywhere, heads bobbed in musical conversation, and bodies moved in sensuous sweeps below kohl-lined eyes.

After lunch we visited the Museum of Tribal Artifacts, the only tourists that Tuesday. The curator met us by the musical instruments and invited us for tea in his office, where a perfectly preserved sandstone block held a corn goddess, identical to Southwest American art. Gujarat's land was similar too, arid and red, spare vegetation. The curator spoke of his expeditions to residual forests in remote regions throughout India, some still unmapped. Places at the mercy of teak and mahogany exporters, of villagers who needed arable land. *The Lonely Planet* guidebook described pockets of indigenous people, Dravidians, but they were said to inhabit small islands off the Eastern mainland.

He insisted they were scattered throughout the subcontinent, and threatened. "We have no surveys," he said. "These people don't know fire, some have no wheel. Forests shelter them," he shook his head. "Sandalwood's endangered, so for the time being some of them are safe." He pulled out a handkerchief, blew his nose. "Prehistoric hibernation, that's what it is. They don't even use time as we know it." He tapped his wrist watch, nodded to the wall clock, shook his head. "Starvation, overpopulation, nuclear annihilation—these are threats to the government. A small group of illiterates who wouldn't vote anyway, not a priority."

He poured our tea, showed us cards he'd made of ancient pictographs. He was a painter, held shows in Tokyo and Paris and Frankfort, to support his anthropology. "They must be documented before they're gone," he said.

There was a one-liner in a guidebook about rural India, that women past menopause are disregarded, considered incomplete humans. We sipped the delicious jasmine despite the heat, happy to be treated well. Then we unzipped our backpacks, found rupees and started to select cards, when his eyes locked on the doorway. Someone had come, a friend, another physician. Perfect, we thought.

But he hustled us out as the man entered, said he'd call at our ashram the next morning with card selections. "Thank you, thank you for coming." No introductions, not even a namaste.

What if time is not human invention? What if it's solid and practical, like food or sleep or death?

At Gandhi's ashram, a dark-skinned, crinkled Harjaran woman swept the street and sidewalks twice a day, cleared tables, stood mute as we passed her to enter the grounds to meditate, study quotes of the Mahatma, "I had always tried to make my wife bend to my wishes," he wrote. "She would firmly refuse to do so and patiently bear the hardships I would inflict in my obstinacy. It was her peaceful opposition that opened my eyes...and rid me of the foolish notion that it is my birthright to rule over her."

The old woman tended the orphans who lived in the ashram, hid beside the kitchen at meals, watching. Our final morning, the museum curator arrived and I thought, an *eye for an eye* so as he sat, I rose and carried a sweet to the old woman. She backed away, hands outstretched to ward me off. Alice, never that confrontational, chose her cards rapidly, appeased the ruffled man. He left. Alice went upstairs to pack, and I sipped coffee, flicked through lecture notes. Soon all the men, manager, waiter, cab drivers, slipped away. It was quiet as a morgue when the crinkle-skinned granny rushed my table. She stuck her face close, shouted, "wayboy," then retreated. I held a banana out, but she shook her head no, closed in again, hot licorice-breath parting my bangs. "Wayboy," she repeated, louder, as if I were deaf. I held up my hands in confusion, the beginning posture of a south Indian dance. She cackled, stepped back, "Means good morning, in Gujarat." She bowed her head above steepled hands, her smile exposed a single tooth. Then she swept her sari close, returned to her corner.

Weeks later, on the steps of Ranthambore Fort, a thousand feet above the wildlife sanctuary/tiger preserve, a small village had fifteen temples and another sweeper. I asked to borrow her broom. She passed me the stubby whisk, no two bristles the same length. I tried to work it seven different ways, away from the steps, flat on the stone, aimed at me, curled my palm around it, held it by two fingers. I never succeeded in moving a single speck.

Even the second year I knew Alice, we were still raw from our first divorces. Outside Hollywood, it was a shame-filled phenomenon in those days, an exception. We spoke by phone from time to time, but one night she called late, upset about a cluster of anti-Semitic incidents in her city, Vancouver. "Canadian reporters are calling it an epidemic," she said. "And our reporters are not alarmists." Canadians in general are not drama junkies. She was afraid for my children, it was the white sheet in the front window, half-a-century earlier: diphtheria, stay away. "No," I said, "It can't be; these are modern times, it's not possible."

Two days later a neighbor's child slammed through the front door, tearing my late-afternoon meditation. She took the stairs two at a time, screaming, "Come quick, Tori's Mom, come. She's getting beat up. They started it, calling her names, a kite," she said. I raced to the block's end where my daughter was sprawled on the green lawn, her cheek scraped, her face smeared in tears. I folded her against me, absorbed her sobs, checked for serious injury, bad cuts, fractures. I soothed her for a minute, then high-tailed it after the gang of girl-thugs, four city blocks ahead. I was thoroughly winded when I caught two, shook their small shoulders until their heads bounced. My daughter healed quickly, as healthy children do, externally. I questioned meditation then, the benefits of pacifism. I questioned everything.

Judson's not Jewish. It's not important now that my children are adults, confident in whatever they believe. It's thirty years after Tori's attack. I could no longer catch the bullies. She knows self-defense; I went to her "graduation," watched her ward off padded "attackers," my stomach churning titillies—butterflies, in Hindi.

And Judson respects women, speaks of his daughter with awe, her character, her brains. She's at Harvard, pre-law, like her dad. It will be different this time, I tell myself. It is different already. He was raised by strong women, a successful businesswoman-mother, and grandmother, who lived in. You can hear admiration in his voice, this man who considers partially-feminine a high compliment.

In Rajasthan, Alice and I toured a fort built in 1411. The roof view, panoramic, revealed a large grassy courtyard filled with young men in white shirts, dark trousers and ties. They were spread over the lawn, typing on black portable Underwoods. We thought it might be a university, but our guide, Sirrender, said, "No, this is the supreme court of Rajasthan. These are lawyers, preparing briefs."

"On the lawn?" Alice asked.

"Ah yes. Sunshine's good for the health, no?" Sirrender's cup was always half-full, except about romance. He suffered an arranged marriage with an uneducated, backward wife. He had a mistress, of course, brought her touring when he could. He complained his wife was so illiterate, she went to the shrine of Ganesh every morning, expecting a miracle.

"She's an ignorant woman," he once said looking at Alice, whose face betrayed her, so he tried hard not to bring up his marriage again. Through long days driving, he spoke of peasants and their superstitions. He pointed out small mud huts stuttering the landscape, where dung paddies dried, so they could be used as fuel. Once started though, he inevitably looped back to his hard life, his wife's flaws. "It's my karma," he sighed. "But my son will have it better."

Alice looked out the window at pendulous nests decorating roadside trees. Her eyes tracked linear young women walking the fields, enormous stacks of dried dung on their heads, hands grasping children or water jugs. "I need to earn money so my boy will be able to choose his own wife. For love," he said, moonstruck. Alice later said she thought he was disgusting, milking us for tips. I wanted to warn him that romance is a fragile system too, but I knew we were older, unhusbanded women, and he would never listen.

Judson's been offered CFO at the bank. The law had been good money for years he said, but its application made him sick. "I loved the elegance of law, the structure, its intent. But it's adversarial, it's all argument. I'm interested in solving problems, that's my gift."

I thought of my daughter, Ariel, then, the time in college I asked what she thought her main talent was. She'd surprised me. "Being a mediator," she'd said fast, like she'd rehearsed it, like she knew, at twenty-three. "I love to negotiate, to help people work things out, together."

I saw, everyone who knew her saw, her abilities in painting and music and dance, in theater. But you never know how others see themselves. With Judson, a trouble-shooter made sense. His mother died by her own hand when he was nineteen. Of course he'd spend his life solving problems. He couldn't bear another catastrophe of that proportion. The first time he mentioned her, his eyes misted. "She would've been a wonderful grandmother, missed all that." He shook his head, for weeks he only mentioned her loss, her never knowing his children.

After we'd dated a month he said, "I went to Europe for a year, after Mom died. Skied. Bummed around. Learned some French, Spanish, a little German. Had sex, lots and lots of sex. Two *menage à trois*." He was playing with me; we were naked on my bed. His brow arched up.

"Was it everything men fantasize, the menage? Was it phenomenal?"

He smiled, leaned over, "Had they been lesbians, it would have been easier. Are you interested? I could teach you to be a lesbian." Then he turned out the light.

"What was it like?" I asked again.

"It was busy, very, very busy."

In subatomic physics there's a recording effect. Observation alters the experiment. Quark spins change, a particle wave inverts, just because it's viewed. Monitoring, perhaps judgment, has an impact on reality.

Working women age at an accelerated pace. Like radioactive elements, we decay faster than normal, more rapidly than our male colleagues. There's never enough time for personal life. Swaths of years blur in childbearing, nursing, working; exercise and nutrition are remote considerations, as is marriage, all too often. Chewing more than half a meal's impossible; bowel movements are squeezed in.

The men Alice and I worked with weren't bad. They led troubled, complex lives too. They experienced identical bedtime efforts to sleep, retinas re-seeing slides, re-thinking borderline lesions that teased even experts. Our eyelids scraped against the night, blotting out freak malformations, a nose on a forehead, an uncovered brain, hearts with huge holes, the rare one, in a tissue-hammock outside the chest. Lifeless bodies reassembled at night, like the *Nutcracker Suite*. We finalized the post mortem, conferenced with the pediatrician and parents, discussed how the child died in antiseptic terms, made a story of events, a fable of comfort. For the family, the clinicians, for ourselves.

Dealing daily with children chewed by cancer, babies suffering enormous tumors, teens dying out of time, for-feited some of our humanity. The emotionless posture of medicine, of pathology in particular, corroded us all.

We were paid well to think hard about hard things. But Alice and I believed, kept hoping, that genuine distance, a blessed detachment, was a skill we would learn, in time. I inhaled self-help books; Alice meditated. We both sought relief in therapy. Nothing worked. Now I wonder we thought it might.

At bi-annual conferences, after a nightcap or two, we promised each other that a kind of peace, a mental safety, was a few more posts, or months, or years away. Our part-ners ascended the medical ladder, moved from the day-to-day bench work to administration, became chairmen.

But timing's everything. The pill was available to us, lucky women. Herpes and AIDS were distant horizons through our thirties. We led full lives, not prudes, and women's salaries increased. Women in all professions fomented change. There were retaliations.

Alice ran for the chair of her department against a close colleague, a friend of many years. An outsider was chosen. "Fair enough," she'd said. But there was a rub: the choice had been made before the contest opened, so the internal competition was divisive and unnecessary. Her partner, the MALE pathologist, was notified a week before the public announcement. The search chairman called his buddy at home, at night, with a "heads-up." He appeared gracious in defeat; Alice looked unraveled. She did receive notification, a form letter, three weeks after everyone else knew.

Our partners never saw the days we cowered on back steps, after a particularly brutal post mortem. Three separate courses of chemotherapy, almost out of danger, and the child got chickenpox, died. No residual leukemia. We cried in private, hugged our knees, imagined the parents.

One Sunday night Alice called, months after a post on a five-year-old. "His body's still here," she said, a whiskey whisper. "His father built him a go-cart for his birthday, insisted he ride it. Story was, the kid was scared. It was a contraption, parts of a wagon, steering wheel from a tractor, four solid rubber tires. The back was cut away for the outboard." Her voice cracked. "Freckles, a face full of freckles. And carrot colored hair. His body wasn't even scratched.

"Go on, the father insisted. The boy wanted to please, but he was small, a careful kind of kid. His father called him *wuss*, so the boy revved the motor, ran into a brick wall, ruptured his liver. All his blood pooled in his abdomen. His skin was so pale I couldn't see the freckles on his forearms. Six months. No one's claimed the body. That's never happened before. He's still in our cooler."

There are arrangements, of course. Every hospital has them. The mom's a teen, there's no money for burial. Fetuses, mostly. Mortuaries perform this community service, provide a common grave for the unclaimed. But not a five year old, never that. "His younger brother saw it happen, for God's sake." Alice said. "His name was Devon."

I tried then, like a therapist or a good friend might, to console her. I listened, recited my own worst post, which occured my first year of residency when my babygirl was still in diapers. That first year of pathology, every death was a horror. I was pregnant with my second and each night I'd get home, I'd scoop my daughter to me, tight, her life, her health, gifts.

Judson understood how adult children remain babies in a parent's brain. How a splintered, perfect hologram lodges, even though the child's grown-up. His face melted the night he recounted the births of each of his children.

Details of labors, the counting of tiny fingers. A man with paternal tenderness is irresistible.

My worst post was a "stat" autopsy. The body had to be transported to Wyoming for services the next day. It was winter, the roads were bad, and I came in right after supper. The baby was emaciated, three months old, so thin he would've qualified as starving, even in India. His mouth and eyes were matched saucers, wide open. I placed a towel over the face, to hide his staring scream, an expression less of terror than surprise. It registered something about time that evades most of us: its intense speed.

His skin "tented," or stuck to itself, wet canvas around a circus-pole. It's a way to estimate dehydration I'd learned as a pediatric intern, how open to run an IV, before the electrolytes come back from the lab.

When I got the autopsy slides back a week later, there were fields of pink collagen between his pancreatic islets, scar tissue obliterating the glands and ducts, which normally secrete digestive enzymes. A thick magenta layer coated his intestines, too. He had starved to death. His distal ileum and colon were distorted by this purply protein. Globules distended glands into microscopic cysts. Cystic fibrosis. In the '70s, doctors did sweat tests when it was suspected. Babies didn't die of it anymore. As I spoke with Alice that night, I still saw his spare blond corona circling his chalky scalp, stark against the steel table, in that chloroxed arena. His astonished eyes, his face, embedded in me.

What if time isn't discrete? What if space, matter, energy and time are really more fluid, interdependent qualities?

Like the stone carvings in Khajuraho, sculpture so vital Alice and I wondered if we shed our skin, if gray writhing stone would lay beneath. These sculpts curl in ecstasy; it's erotic to simply view them. Faces, postures, orgasms, union with the divine. These were why I was in India. Alice came to deepen spiritual connections. She has unwavering faith that good will result from correct behavior, from right effort. She doesn't share my delight in the ups and downs of life; cataclysms that stimulate me. Some years I think I need them to prove I'm still alive. Perhaps it's temperament, or perhaps she's trained herself calm. She nourishes everyone else's hungers as if she were not the main actor in her life; a selflessness I admire, but will never match.

Americans rarely tour Khajuraho, and those who come, stay outside. The temple interiors are poorly lit, no real windows, no electricity. There are high slits in the masonry, a few flickering candles, and steepled ceilings that are almost black. Entrances are forbidding too, on top of multi-storied steep stone steps. We lost count at seventy. A shy young man guided us, carried his bible, offered convoluted religious explanations for the exterior carvings. He never went inside. "See the man's finger touching the woman's spine," he asked, ignoring the enormous penis perforating her. "He's circulating her energy so it properly ascends through her chakras."

The centerpiece of each temple was a huge circular stone, with a carved meatus. Even ill-lit, there was no mistaking each lingum, or the space on the floor in front of it, lipped and voluptuous, a yoni. Pieces were torn away in some temples, just as lower, exterior statues missed genitals or breasts. We toured three interiors before Alice recognized the ceilings were moving. Thousands of bats wriggled above us.

Overnight in Khajuraho, we attended a service at a functional temple adjacent to the historic grounds. Loud parishioners circled, danced, and swooned around a huge black lingum. Men and women approached the sculpt, twenty feet in diameter, two stories high, kissed their hands, touched their genitals, fell on their knees, touched the lingum again. Their worship made intuitive sense to me. During college I'd sampled many denominations, studied comparative religion for three semesters. I never found the combination of ceremony and open-heart that resonated, until India. I'd been raised Catholic, left that in high school, converted to Judaism in medical school to please my first husband. I was rule-numb, appalled at wrathful gods, felt somewhat cheated because there were no goddesses. In a strange land, in a language I didn't begin to understand, fertility worship struck me as real, as universal as hope.

Like Judson. Fleshy love, primitive, tangible, absorbing. I never expected this again. Wasn't sure I wanted it. Periodically, I'd panic. I called him one day at work, early in our romance. "You won't leave me, will you?" I asked. "This isn't real, is it?" I abandoned all medical training. *Ask only open-ended questions. Never frame a question with a negative. Always, always watch for body language; the body doesn't lie.* But I'd phoned him.

"If I love you and I'm behind you, I'll never leave you," he said. No hesitation. "And I do love you, but you know that," as if reassuring a child.

Einstein said there were only two things that were infinite, space-time, that flimsy expanse into which everything's spreading since the big bang, and human ignorance.

Our final Indian destination was Varanarsi, Benares under the British; the longest continuously inhabited city on the planet. It smelled true. It was wildly crowded, the air fetid, the Ganges filthy. We arrived the day before Duvali, the most important holiday in the Indian calendar, a collective Christmas, New Years, Thanksgiving and Fourth of July. We'd scheduled a car and driver to take us to Sarnath, where Buddha found enlightenment under the Bodi tree. The morning of Duvali we were to rise early and witness sunrise on the Ganges. At the hotel, our chief guide called from Delhi to tell us there would be no Sarnath. There were no cabs or drivers available. "So sorry, Duvali," he said and Alice looked deflated. I took the phone and became a New Yorker again, insisting, arguing, ranting until he said, "Tomorrow, perhaps day after tomorrow."

We napped before supper, the hour in the crowds had sapped us. It had been a long, wonderful trip, but even great times deplete us now, energy has strict, stingy limits.

In the morning we rose to another phone call. It was Sirrender again, from Delhi. "Please to tell you, there will be a driver at two. Please to remind the madams, not to go out this morning. Tomorrow morning, we will arrange a driver to the Ganga. Not safe for madams to go out this morning. But this afternoon, a driver. Thank you."

"Why?" I asked. "Are the crowds dangerous? They're celebrating New Year, no?"

"Well yes, Madame," and a long pause, "but there is to be an eclipse."

"Marvelous," I said. He has a cell phone, a laptop; it's his wife who's superstitious.

"No, no Madame. You are my responsibilities. It is very inauspicious."

"Well all right," I said, crossing my fingers. "Thanks. Mr. Guphta, at two then. We'll be waiting in the lobby."

We dressed quickly in the dark, hired a rickshaw and arrived near the mobbed ghat, the bank of the Ganges, before dawn. Winding streets to the river were lined by a sinuous path of ground-level beggars, mostly reclining, faces half hidden in bandages. There were lepers, amputees, and paralytics who exposed their wounds as we passed. They extended hands, laced with sores, fingers missing. There was a sacred cow lying among them, a hoof half-eaten away. I closed my eyes and saw *Mycobacterium leprae*, close relative of tuberculosis, a beaded, carmine organism, glistening refractive on a slide set I'd studied for boards. Alice and I pulled kerchiefs over our mouths, the foulness of open sewers and sores mixed with the surfeit of humanity. The sun was barely up as throngs of people milled along the river, stripped to their waists or totally; strangers, side by side in the filthy water, slopping brown liquid over their bodies and heads. Many held their mouths open to swallow holiness. We were astonished, not so much by the lack of modesty in a country that considers shoulder exposure pornographic, but by the solemnity. Families carried small brass pots and pitchers of river water up the ghat, sipping and pouring it over one another as they caught their breath at the top of the steep stone steps.

The air cloaked us as we walked back up to the street crowds. The sun slid behind the moon. Light and shadow rearranged space. Darkness silenced everyone.

The crowd thinned, and for a full thirty minutes, everything suspended. We all stepped out of time.

Back at the hotel we took another nap. It was only eleven a.m. when Sirrender called, "So sorry Madams. No transportation. A holiday. So, so sorry. Tomorrow, early. I promise. Yes, yes, my word."

That evening we asked the concierge for a restaurant, away from the hotel, and he sent us to a small place on a barren block, close. The parking lot was huge, well lit, empty. It was only seven-thirty, and we thought maybe they adhered to European dining time. Inside there were no customers either. The lighting was extremely dim. The waiter hurried with glasses of water and menus.

We ordered hot food and bottled water as our eyes adjusted. Alice saw it first, pointed to the walls. The wallpaper moved. We shared this Kafka moment, insects everywhere. Armies crawled the walls. We looked at the table, nothing. "I hope you wore socks with your Birks," Alice said, as tiny roaches, or worse, skittered over my instep.

I stamped my feet, keeping time to hallucinatory music. The food arrived, steaming platters which in seconds, were covered by flying roaches, buzzing vectors. We looked at each other and I signaled the waiter for the check; but when he came, Alice indicated the bugs, blackening all the platters. In a country of Hindus and Jains, he'd understand vegetarianism. He nodded, vanished into a back room.

"He's going to get DDT and spray us," I said, beginning to laugh at the joke the concierge had played.

"Don't be ridiculous," Alice said. "It's been banned internationally for decades." She fanned the rice, almost succeeded in ridding it of its chitinous cover, waving her hands like I blessed Sabbath candles, Friday nights.

He returned with a huge DDT canister, the metal pump type Nana used. Clouds of insecticide covered our food, our faces, our clothes, before we could object. Alice shrugged; we paid and left. We showered for half an hour apiece at the hotel, even though the water ran frigid. We could have saved resources, scrubbed each other's skin, but I would never suggest that.

The next morning, Mr. Ghupta arrived before sunrise. He wore a clean pressed shirt, shiny slacks, and the most enormous ear hair, ever. Two curling black tufts sprouted symmetrically, skimmed each shoulder, and curled up to touch his temples. It had to be some genetic oddity, but neither of us knew its name. We barely breathed in the rear of the cab. I disabled the flash, hoped to document the black circular silhouettes, backlit by the windshield.

We got to the Ganges and entered a small rickety boat, as dawn pinked the sky. Our skinny seven-year-old "oarsman" rowed through hundreds of tiny floating oil lamps, lit for separate souls. We passed two crematoria which burned wood pyres, night and day. The boatsman said photography of them was prohibited; he would be banned from the river. "Cremation is only for adults," he said. "Their sins need to be burned away, their ashes purified, returned to mother river. Children under five are slipped into the water at night. They don't need cremation," his head rocked from side to side, "too young to sin," he smiled, both front teeth missing.

On a top step, far from the crowds, a lean giant, white hair wrapped around his skull like a huge turban, pulled a ram's horn from his tunic, blew it, hollow, melancholy. The sound penetrated, a universal ohm, crossed the inky river to the waiting sun, which rose, obediently. A huge orange ball cinnamoned the distant bank. I turned to Alice, "I bet this is where our high holy day rituals began. The shofar's a ram's horn too, blown to announce sundown on Rosh Hashanah, Yom Kippur."

I started to tell this to Judson, how we could share one another's family celebrations, create new history, our own. By the time I thought to say this though, he'd entered panic.

What if time is different from the proposed continuum, that two-dimensional cartoon aired periodically on PBS diagramming the fourth dimension, which our senses cannot grasp. A representation of Einstein's thoughts, as if the rest of us could follow him into the folding, gyrating "fourth." We all know geometry, lines, and height, width, curves even, see

*them, feel them, walk on them. And we know space, the ether
that separates us; the stops that makes sentences work. But
time...as part of that space, that's not intuitive.*

In 1982, at a conference near Santa Monica, Alice and
I shared a berth on the *QEII*. The sea was pitted with oil
rigs pumping like duck-in-the-cup toys. Lead-weighted
bellies bobbed in exaggerated arcs, like women beating
clothes on river banks throughout India. In California, we
rehearsed our papers to each other, caught up on recent
lovers. It was years after our first divorces; I was mad
about Lamar, a pilot, a high-and-bye man who wooed me
hard, then flew away. Alice had just exited a long-term
live-in relationship with a bus driver, and we tried to
think of ties between transportation and pathology, but
it was the pathology of the men that glued us.

Her honey and companion for her thirties insisted
he didn't want children. Alice relinquished that dream
for the security of him. When she discovered his affair,
she was crushed. He invited her to their too-hasty wedding, expected, probably, that she'd offer to host the baby
shower. I was more outraged than she. Time heals everything, Nana used to say at childhood disappointments.
I had no patience for that homily when I was young; I'm
still not a believer.

In California, Alice meditated twice a day. I'd never
gotten to that point of discipline, or faith. That amount
of being still in prayer moved awfully close to formaldehyde for me. But I saw the incredible goodness that grew
in her, became cellular in age, an art form. And of course,
I wanted that.

Alice reminded me that calm would probably grate my
core; that something in me craved cayenne and jalapeños
and vinegar. Besides, my new romance was still perfect.
Even its intermittent quality was a plus: alone-time to
tend the children, a tense career, then the bite and excitement of Lamar, returned.

Alice was to teach a half-day seminar, so I spent Saturday driving the coast with another long-time friend,
Nola, a character actress. I'd wanted them to meet for
dinner, but Alice had man-plans, the brother of an old

flame. Nola invited me to a party Saturday night, and I stayed over, met her girls again, grown women now. They were toddlers when we lived near each other in Denver, as young mothers. I didn't leave Nola's number for Alice, or at the ship, because Alice had thought she might spend the night with her date. So I'd called home, left Nola's number there; my children were fine. I forgot home as Nola and I drove the freeway south, criss-crossing beneath the shadow of one of California's last free condors. A huge, black, solitary raptor rode thermals for hours, ignorant that as a species, it was almost extinct. Or maybe that's why it soared.

We stopped periodically to walk the beach, especially where it was deserted. It was a double-dip day for my life-list because, by late afternoon, I'd seen an oystercatcher too. Tall, jet-black, it had an elongate red bill. We saw it choose a mollusk, then drop the shell over and over on a rock until it finally opened to pearl-gray muscle.

The call from my pilot came in the morning, before Alice was up. "She was here last night," she told him. "No, I have no idea why she didn't answer. Maybe they gave you the wrong room. Maybe she was going to the bathroom. Did you leave a message for her to call back?" Alice got up and began pacing, the phone against her ear. "I don't understand why you're so upset. She's loyal, deeply in love with you. She's spent half the time here, talking about you. You're a very lucky man. Yes, I'll have her call."

By the time I got back, mid-morning, Alice was beside herself. "He sounds fearfully jealous. Obsessive. How stable is he? He sounds like poison." I should have asked about antidotes right then.

"Oh, no, he's normal," I said, "just melodramatic. And it's sort of flattering he's so crazy about me." Motherhood breeds a strange kind of craving for protection, a need to feel safe in someone's attention and physicality, wrapped, the way you try to safeguard your children. In many ways his jealousy felt like an invisible insurance policy. I admit it sounds sketchy for a feminist, sounds more like cave-woman-think or girl-fantasies from the '50s. Young Canadian women may have been raised on autonomy and heroines, but in the U.S., our diet was dependence.

When I think *love*, I think: jangled nerves, dark chocolate, crashing, chemical encounters, heightened life, need. And I have gladly, repeatedly, immersed myself in it, every chance I get. Like an addict. Like Judson. We could have been thirteen, it was that hot. All caution, all previous lessons, every measured response, trashed.

This worship of romance, or lust, will need a wooden stake to stop. Even during my bout with cancer and the radical surgery, the smarmy shot-gun divorce from my wild pilot, my body hungered for him. A philanderer who stole a great deal of my money, I still wanted him. But I got lucky. During my hospitalization he called Alice to enlist her help. He referred to my history of mental illness. Lamar didn't know we shared this shame, and said I'd taken leave of my senses again. "Maybe it's the anesthesia," he said. "Or the pain meds, but she's barring me from the hospital. I'm her husband," he bellowed. "I have rights." And God bless Alice, she dug deep, hurled invectives I didn't know she knew.

There are dissenting doubters in science who suggest maybe, just maybe, the world didn't begin in a bang. Maybe all matter didn't originate at once, streaming away from itself into void. After all, where did void come from? Maybe the theory that the future will run out of spreadability, space and matter will implode again, is just hypothesis, could be wrong.

Alice cut her hair. So have I. The cut versions are peppered gray. We bought identical silver filigree barrettes in Agra to remind ourselves we could regrow our hair, and to have something exquisite from the home of the Taj. We were both speechless before this memorial to love. A mughal risked ridicule, his entire kingdom, and spent the last twenty years of his life in prison to build a mausoleum for one woman. Not his first or last wife, but the one he loved. She died in childbirth with their nineteenth son, at thirty-seven.

The building was planned so no cityscape would ever be close enough for visual reference. An architect's trick; the structure backs on the Yamuna River, wide, brown, serpentine, where women slap crimson and saffron saris against flat rocks. The memorial is flanked by four minarets, one per corner, which slope ninety-three degrees away from the marble structure, just off-perpendicular. This provides optical symmetry, so as you approach the treasure, snap your photos, the façade remains a constant distance in front, frozen. Only the two or three final steps brings you close enough to be quite suddenly, dwarfed.

In Agra one evening, we left our hotel without Sirrender. We were a little scared, but our journey was almost over, and we wanted unfiltered India. A rickshaw brought us to dense street markets with locals. I bought tiny gold earrings with intricate screw backs for a hundred rupees, brass pots for pens, three rupees apiece. A white-coated, bearded man smoked in a doorway; the storefront looked pharmaceutical. We nodded, told him we were doctors from North America, asked if we could look.

"This is my office," he said. "Come in, come in."

We told him we'd lectured at All India Medical College in Delhi, and he said, "Madras," tapping his chest. A locked cabinet held drugs on the left side of a small main room. Two tiny alcoves behind that were separated by thin white curtains. Each back "room" had a narrow examining table, a sphygmomanometer, a scale, and steel cabinets with sutures, gauze, plaster. Old crutches leaned against one wall which housed a sterilizer. In a niche there were three sets of forceps, and an ancient vacuum extractor. The instruments were clean, but the equipment looked like a field hospital, circa World War I.

I asked about birth control, if he performed abortions, and all color drained from his face. "The Jains are very active here," he said. "All life is precious. We do not perform abortions." He shook his head vigorously, wagged his finger. I blushed, thanked him for his time, brought my palms together in namaste. He relaxed then, and showed us a shelf of Aryvedic herbs, tapped each bottle with a foreign name, then defined a familiar disease. As we turned to leave, Alice said, "D&Cs then, do you perform D&Cs?"

"Oh, yes, yes." His head wobbled back and forth. "Very necessary. We do many every day, we are doing many."

Next door there was a cosmetic shop, and I purchased small pots of pigment for Tori as Alice slipped back to the clinic, made a substantial donation.

The next day we returned to the Taj before sunrise, made four separate day-trips, and another at dusk. The marble morphed in different light, blue before dawn, dove-gray late morning, white in full sun, then pink, salmon at sundown. As we circled the exterior around eleven a.m., women on the riverbank stacked wet wash on their heads, and immediately and forever, Alice and I thought differently about hard work. We'd believed we were weary, years of over-long days, when life pressed like a barium swallow, dense opaque sludge, no nourishment. We'd spent years learning techniques, studying constantly, so we'd know the latest sub-categorizations for tumors. We read medical journals, not *Good Housekeeping*, wrote chapters and papers, rare friendly letters. Sunny afternoons we did frozen sections, attended conferences, reviewed cases with residents, interns, clinicians. Our bodies grew dusty with disuse. Suborbital shadows circled our eyes, decades of indentations from microscope eyepieces. Our forearms splayed from resting beside the scope all those years. That skin's sprayed with liver spots now. Goose bumps used to rise there, long ago, when we were deeply moved, or fearful. What can we possibly fear now? Retribution for life choices? Time's too short for that.

Age has one advantage, though, you can never predict when deep affection will swivel you in a new dimension. Alice is immersed in fabric design now, and I'm wild about writing. We also know that, although there may be days you want to, you will not die of heartbreak. It isn't like Hemingway insisted, because you're stronger in the broken place. It's because you're grateful for life, for whatever's left.

For her birthday this year I wrote Alice a long letter, by hand, some about him, about my new hymn. History, already.

I reminisced about that Breckenridge streamside, de-cades back. The greybrown dipper that bobbed along stones, dove into the swirling water. How it swam below the surface as Alice and I entered each other's lives, air bubbles adhering to its feathers, wings folded back. Alice had knelt beside that stream, a thing neither of us can do today. She unclasped her hair, let it slither down her back. Her hands did a sensuous dance then, which I've watched for years, braiding, coiling, combing, fastening. The dipper emerged, shook itself on the flat, hot rock, the way she would step from the shower at anonymous Hiltons, in everycity, steam haloing her body, the cello shaped-torso, gleaming, alive, beautiful. I never let her see me look.

That first riveting connection with Alice is engraved, the way she squinted against the sun, cupped her hands to shade her eyes, watched me watch the bird. We did nothing but enjoy nature then. Time will not change us that much, I thought. We'll always be able to finish each other's sentences, even in age. We'll have years of history, work-related conversations, syncopated letters, long distance calls.

We were symphonies once, Alice; rosined strings of men slipped through our hands, resting briefly between breasts and thighs. Maybe not that many, maybe none briefly enough.

During your last phone call, you spoke of an occasional longing, but you said you don't really miss men. "Waking dreams," you called them. You've folded yourself closed against those bitter breakfasts, tantrums and tears. Your body curves a little now, like a sideways smile.

Part of me envies your detachment, but my body still wants. For years at a time, I'd leave one shoulder unwashed all day, stippled with the scent of Lamar. As I write this, I thumb through old photographs, faint pictures of men, my children, small and technicolor, everything fading, even the records of our trips, of us, young and radiant, expecting the world.

Memory is so much longer than truth. In my letter, I remind Alice of the founding mother of pediatric pathology, Edith Potter, who turned from the morgue in age, like we are beginning to. She moved to clean earth and orchids, nourished her eighties and nineties studying and categorizing epiphytes, published a delicious compendium on them at ninety-six. Hard to believe it was over a quarter century ago that we strolled through fallen leaves with the intention of becoming competent professionals; ignorant of how we'd stumbled through some spatial curl, how our lives would stay twined.

Women in medicine in the '60s and '70s had to be committed. Alice and I were dedicated to our first husbands, determined to be good wives as well as good doctors. We went to the cities our men chose, cobbled our training around theirs. These men were the eccentrics, I see that now, wed to career-oriented, aggressive women. They encouraged and supported our aspirations, at least in public. We believed they understood equality, we needed to believe they believed in us.

Militant, Judson said, when I told him how my first baby was born in my internship; that I'd returned to work a month after delivery. His negative take startled me. What could he know of doctoring, or of biologic mothering?

Each first husband lost interest eventually, and we were confounded. We danced our ardor, wild women, idiots, which got each of us committed to asylums, by them, almost simultaneously.

"Trainer wheels for a first bike," Alice once said of that marriage. "An experiment, like hanging wheels off my hips. I rode into medicine, thought he'd balance me, fell anyway. Those protrusions were dead weight, no cushion at all."

After our releases from nuthouses, we each spent years in Freudian infernos; sessions squeezed between hours at the scope and housekeeping, grocery shopping, cooking, scanning slides for definitive malignant features. Our stat reading days are over, but the dipping continues, the clock grinds, the child rests in deep artificial sleep, as a part of him, a lower leg, a quarter of a liver, a region of spinal cord, shines in the OR light. And what is malignant rests on a new pathologist's say-so, on something as flimsy as someone's word.

The nervous beating of that streamside dipper measured time with its obsessive ticking tail, like the second hand of the watch when we dipped a slide for sixty seconds in the ammonia bath, after the hematoxylin, locking cobalt into nuclei. Cell centers so thick in certain tumors, you could hold the slide to light, make your call by naked eye alone, that blue. The pit formed in the stomach then, the mitotic rate was astronomical: the limb would be lost, or the whole child.

It would be hopeful to think time-space is cyclic, like women's lives, the women's movement. I was an early feminist, subscribed to *MS* when Gloria Steinem still ran it. I paraded the streets of Denver in a white dress, sometimes in my white coat, marching for the Equal Rights Amendment. Stories in her magazine moved me deeply. I still remember two. The first was by a South African towns-woman who so loved her best friend, a recent widow, that she loaned her husband to the neighbor as a birthday gift. Their poverty was so grim, material gifts were impossible. The generous woman baby-sat both sets of children that night. It was simply written, the gesture open and pure; it sounded normal to me.

The second story involved old women in nursing homes, in their seventies and eighties, still riffled by desire. They exercised and read books, gardened and gossiped, but their lives were sterile. The concept of that much idleness and isolation was as remote as the elliptical orbit of Io around Jupiter. I was Tori's age then, mid-thirties.

The women in the piece were all heterosexuals, widows, who hugged freely, as women do. In age they turned to one another for touch. At first it was circumspect; chaste pecks on the cheeks at holidays, an arm around a shoulder during sadness. But the affections grew, intimacy developed while they weren't looking. I remember clipping the article, considered sending it to my mother for Mother's Day. But the more I thought about it, the less appropriate it seemed. And then Dad outlived her by years.

I've always loved the company of women, had rare, intermittent attractions. "Loving a woman," a roommate at a writer's conference once confided, "is easy, so easy. First of all, there's the emotional connection. You never misread a woman. And the physical, you've got the same equipment." Easy for her I thought, I'm a mother. She continued. "It's like a secret handshake, a society housed in you since birth. Just dormant."

I never thought seriously about this, until India. Our overnight accommodations in Ranthambore park were a shared bed in a converted Maharaja's hunting lodge. In the middle of the night, I awoke to find my arm around Alice's waist. The next night her hand crawled over my shoulder. We peeled apart, whoever woke first, and we never spoke of it, of course. Once, when she visited me right after my cancer surgery, her hand reached under the table to pet my dog. It was my knee she stroked, through thick surgical stockings, before she realized there were no ears, no wet nose. She reddened then, over-apologized. I was sorry I hadn't said anything, but only because it embarrassed her.

I've known a few women who are "bi," enough to make me rethink, perhaps broader orientation is expansive.

Recent astronomical observers insist that less than four percent of the universe is visible. One-third of everything is dark matter; two-thirds, energy humans cannot see or measure. We extrapolate how things in space behave from earth-observations, knowledge of a small fraction of reality. All those years studying medicine, I believed chemistry, physics, and mathematics were built on fact. Medicine might be part art, but not the hard sciences. What if everything solid we've ever learned is fluctuating, morphable, illusion?

In Varanarsi Alice joked, behind her handkerchiefed nose, that we'd done the childhood game, and began counting fingers. We'd each had our rich men, poor men, beggarmen, and I'd even had a thief. We'd had doctors and lawyers, were only missing chiefs. "Could we substitute a sitar player?" she'd asked, pulling her left ring finger back.

Alice's final fling was a lawyer, head of his own firm, successful, father of teens, divorced five years. Perfect, I thought. Carl promised that elusive brass ring after a few months: a wedding. All red lights muted. I was ecstatic for her. But then it was postponed, and we were still attending meetings, sharing a room. So I overheard her, too many nights, encourage him to do what he needed. Office tensions mounted, he spiraled into depression. She supported this mid-life crisis, paid therapy, paid for private schools for his children.

It was on the DC trip, Alice mentioned Gandhi's advice on celibacy; how she'd found it pivotal in her own spiritual growth.

"What?" I'd asked.

"Being asexual. It pens energy, so you can redirect it to creative work." She was deep in the final revision of her second textbook, but I picked that scab until she confessed they hadn't had sex in years. "He no longer finds me attractive. But that's okay," she insisted as I wailed, my one-eighth Irish ancestry filling the room. I was afraid to ask about other practices the Mahatma used, cleansing enemas for close friends, starvation fasts for weeks.

When Carl finally left, reaming Alice of even more money and a horse ranch, I tried to console her. "You'll pour back into yourself again," I said. But even speaking those words sounded empty.

Like Judson's promises, early, flung life-rafts. "I'll never make love with you unless we're connected," he'd said, when I hadn't asked for anything.

The night we drove back from his California vacation, we were both exhausted by the week of sun and surf and sex. We'd broken camp that morning, drove to his boyhood home on alkali flats, where they test-piloted jets. We drove on through the night until two a.m. The motel was outside Reno, dark, undistinguished. I barely brushed my teeth, lay down, fell asleep. He began then, a gentle prodding, loving me once more, a very concrete connection.

In hindsight, I should've listened to my sister. "Why would you fly to California and surprise him?" she scolded. "Leave it alone. Remember absence and the heart?"

Even Tori had cautioned, "Don't burn it all out in a month, Ma."

But there were his yearning calls, five, six, seven hours a day, everyday. Across Colorado, Utah, Nevada, and through California. Talking, talking, upgrading his cellphone plan five times. We shared childhood intimacies, adult experiences we'd kept secret for decades. And when he got to the beach, he begged me to join him. I went. That week of reptilian love cured all residual longing for my second ex, a desire that had plagued me through a dozen years of therapy. Five weeks of Judson: done.

On the interminable drive back, his life began to un-hinge. He'd accepted the CFO position before the trip, but now there was to be an investigation, an audit. And, each of his children had a Daddy-crisis. He never once said anyone was with him in the car when he spoke to them. Why then, when we were both almost sick with exhaus-tion, when we would sleep only a few hours anyway, why did he make love and resurrect that early promise?

At my condo entrance on Sunday night, cool as any surfer dude, Judson clasped my hand, shook it. "Thank you for coming, and being with me." As if I were a baby sitter.

Two weeks later, we had a final supper. He discussed his handball game for two hours. A little about his job, the increased pressures, how his youngest decided not to stay with his mom, not even half-time. How he was too damaged to be in a relationship. How wonderful I was. How I deserved better, deserved a partner who could be there for me.

Come on, I almost screamed, I'm a writer. You can't use sitcom dialogue. But what I said was different. "Okay then, let's kick back to Platonic for a few months, until things settle. I single-raised three children the best part of fifteen years. I know what it's like to be drawn and quartered." I did not say how exceptional this love was. That I'd dated others since my last husband, had tried to fall in love, safely, using logic and character. But this is not how it goes, not really. The body has its own agenda, moves in its own time frame, to its own thrum. Only he was done.

When he said it, words weren't necessary. He'd been limping all evening, an old back injury hit during hand-ball. I'd reached to massage him, but his body recoiled.

Maybe he feared I'd change my mind someday; moth-ers do that. Or maybe he was being kind, saw we couldn't possibly make it, knew in six months, or three years, his departure might kill me.

That night was an eternity of sleeplessness. I dialed his number over and over, hung up before speaking; a stalking kind of grief. At first light, that smoldering gray-blue, I called, left a witch's message. "I need your HIV results. I need my books back. And you don't know me. You said we moved too fast, you weren't in a position to commit. You said I felt the same, you knew I did. What happened was simple: we were attracted to each other." Strong force.

"You were wrong. You don't know how I feel. I do love you. I'm old enough to know when I'm in love. And serenading me with that Matchbox Twenty song, *Hand me Down*. You made me believe the lyrics. *It's all right, lay your troubles down, I'm with you now.* You made promises I'd never asked for, a future of caring, wild lovemaking, a home together. It was love, not dumb animal attraction." I was sobbing by the time I hung up.

Astronomers insist the universe is expanding at ever increasing speed. Authorities say empty space contains mysterious energy that pushes things apart. Stars, galaxies, friends, even lovers, fly from each other.

The same weekend Judson ended things, a minor miracle occurred. Months before, I'd scheduled a meditation retreat with Thich Nat Hahn for that Sunday. I didn't think I'd be able to sit through it. Saturday I'd wandered the malls in shades, with one of those crying headaches I hadn't had in years. I'd called every sympathetic woman friend I knew, for commiseration, until I couldn't bear to speak or listen any longer. I postponed telling my sister. She was going to gloat. When I'd first whispered about the affair, she'd said, "Well, we'll see how long this lasts."

Six weeks, by threads. But she was sympathetic. Midnight Saturday though, I wondered if I'd made it all up, the intensity, the proclamations of love, the bliss. Was it purely physical? He'd played my body like a stringed instrument; but there were those hours of conversation, in person, and by phone. Somewhere in Nevada, he had pulled to the side of the road and wept over his mother's death. He said he'd never cried about her all those years. He confided how his first wife wielded his suicide-guilt, like a weapon at the end. How his second wife tried to pit him against his son, how he'd warned her; how she hadn't stopped.

I listened to feelings he'd never shared before. I held him until the pain emptied.

It was Alice who made me laugh. *Well*, she said, *at least you've completed the program. CFO is a chief after all, even if it's only finances.*

I slept fitfully Saturday night, floated in and out, dreamed of visiting my father's mother, in the nursing home.

"What's it like Grandma?" I'd asked, the final time I actually saw her. The rest of the family went to lunch, my sister and parents, my aunt, who all knew she was senile.

"Somedays, for hours at a time, I'm sixteen again. My skin's new, my waist is small, I dance. Or I'm pregnant and nursing. It's beautiful," she said, tears runneled her cheeks. "Quite suddenly, on accident, I'm old. A time mistake." She laughed then, a croaky sound shook her body. She swiveled her head around anxiously, pulled a cigarette from her pocket. I lit it, guided it to crinkled lips; the end fired red.

The Buddhist retreat began with groupies chanting, issuing orders. "Sit down. Close your eyes. Empty your mind." I gave myself permission to leave, just as Thich Nat Hahn entered. Something beatific filled the room. I smelled violets. It was as peaceful as the last afternoon with Grandma. Sun slanting over us, we sat silent, my palm cupped below her cigarette, catching ashes. And then, I was forgiving Judson during the meditation, composing the e-mail I sent later that night, thanking him for the good times, telling him to ignore my phone message, wishing him well. Which me was me?

Maybe the universe has a dichotomous structure. Maybe it does move in waves, like an accordion, in and out, matter/non-matter, time/notime. Maybe it's a helix, now we see each other, age, rotate, dream each other young, back peddle, pulse forward. Maybe it's irrelevant where we really are along the curve. Maybe it only matters that we are kind.

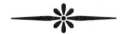

Late July 1991, I had a cone biopsy before my hysterectomy for cancer. A week later I picked the slides up to take to the surgeon. My colleague asked if I wanted to review them first. I did and I didn't. I was weak, used my hands to lower my body into the chair at the double-headed scope. "I really don't know adult pathology," I began. "I'm not sure I'd recognize adenocarcino—holy shit, are those in my body?"

My left hand adjusted the fine focus and a sea of dark blue cells, dividing and spreading over normal tissue, came into perfect clarity.

I faint at my first everything in medical school.
First cadaver.
First surgery.
First autopsy.
Well not everything, not the first lecture.
I even blow the tour, the first day.

The tour's really a test. We're in, MCAT scores high enough, first semester tuition paid. Our entire freshman class files into the sub-basement, bound together tight as a brownie troop. The space is gigantic, our footsteps echo, and it's so cold we all feel small. We huddle at the edge of an auditorium-sized meat-locker in one of Philadelphia's five medical schools, in a riot quadrant of the city. Autumn, 1964. We wear short white-coats, to advertise we're only students. We all live close to the school, in the ghetto, where police line rooftops with strobe lights and machine guns every night. It is hot, still Indian summer outside, but in the basement, it's so frigid we flap our arms, open and close fists, stamp our feet to beat back the chill. Our teeth chatter so we can hardly hear the instructor.

My classmate's breaths form little white clouds, like thought bubbles in comic books. It's several minutes before any of us notice the overhead trolley, a sinuous steel ceiling track, like the retrieval runner in an enormous dry-cleaner. The instructor pushes a button, and a ratcheted metallic movement begins, clacking like Dad's "O" gauge trains at Christmas. The air is brittle glass. There are no colorful dresses or navy suits circling; instead, huge, plastic-wrapped mannequins sway in a bizarre dance, with no clear beat. Our breath fogs the amorphous figures who rotate above us. An exceedingly long minute passes.

This is where they store cadavers. Each body is clasped behind the ears by huge, shiny calipers, each skull indents by what could be old fashioned ice tongs, from my childhood, Catskill summers. Mother and I stayed upstate with her parents in the cool mountains during July and August. Dad tutored summer school in the city. My Nana and Pop-Pop rented a small cottage, outhouse, water pump, tin-lined ice-box. The iceman came Monday and Thursday, his pickup bed covered with a tarp. He moved huge clear blocks from the sawdust into our kitchen. His ice pick punched hard staccato cracks as he split our portion. He carried the ice inside with tongs, his face crimson, making subsonic grunts. His biceps bunched then, almost split his shirt, and stiff dark hair on his forearms stood at attention, like I do now, in the doorway. The medical tongs indent skin, but don't pierce it. The bodies are almost silver, rigid glaciers in their transparent comforters. The room is deliberately ill-lit. The cadavers continue their waltz, but several of us hear only a few more bars, before we grab the door sill, and "fall out," Philadelphia's euphemism for fainting.

The first surgery I witness is a hysterectomy, months later. My fiancé arranges this extravagant gift for our winter break. We're to watch his uncle-gynecologist operate. Actually, my boyfriend will assist. My classmates are green. I'm in love, in medical school, we're planning our wedding, crocuses are just below ground, waiting for snowmelt. His uncle peels the skin back, ivory, and soft as cream. This is years before music is standard in the OR, so the only sounds are suction, requests for instruments, and the wheeze of the breathing apparatus.

My mother had a hysterectomy when I was a senior in high school. She was pale and sad that whole year, so I had to do housekeeping, everybody's laundry, grocery shopping, make supper. She kept talking about not wanting to live. He cuts a thick yellow layer of fat that has stringy white divisions between the grease. As the peritoneum opens, jellied pink viscera squeeze in front of my eyes, snaky tan-gray intestines, the fuchsia tip of a spleen, an edge of liver, maroon like raw liver, followed by a kaleidoscope of multi-hued dots, then black. Next I know, I'm on my back, braced by an aroma of coffee. A deep voice I don't recognize booms from green scrubs, *That always happens first time out. Here, have some joe.* He hands me a cup, I ease up on my elbow, sip carefully. I scald my tongue anyway. I feel the pulse in my throat, behind my eyes; my cheeks flush. I apologize, stretch my arms hard overhead, get up, stomp my feet, and insist on returning through the swinging doors. The first hit of aromatic anesthesia brings neon lights and darkness again. This time I regroup longer, walk the halls as instructed, put on a fresh gown and mask, re-enter.

My fiancé doesn't look up. *You're going to have to learn detachment,* he says. He's a junior. I think, right. The belly's splayed open, her uterus glistens, the shape of a steer-skull, clamped by instruments. Thin threads string from each end, blooming to anemones in harsh OR light. She's being eviscerated by my husband-to-be. He tugs retractors and toothed forceps, pulls her organs up and out. All the blood vessels are ligated with black silk, like a belly full of braids. The diseased uterus is not mine, but it could be.

In high school, when I visited mother after surgery, she was barely distinguishable from the sheets. Her lips were parched and white as grade-school paste. My father roamed the halls then, joked with nurses, avoided her room. I wiped her forehead and her eyes followed me, as though she wanted to say something, didn't know where to start. Years before, I'd vowed never to marry anyone who would say, *Over my dead body*, if I wanted to try something new, like Dad had with Mom. *For my birthday I want to apply to college, Milton.* She was turning forty. *I want to teach. I don't think I'm too old, do you? I'm not too old.* He roared through our thin walls, *No wife of mine works outside this house. Not while I breathe.* I put my fingers in my ears then, and later, in the basement, iced and pierced both earlobes. I wanted a reminder to put my own holes in my head.

But this hysterectomy is not my mother's; it's a stranger's. And now I'm in love, a multifaceted emotion, like a diamond. A silly symbol my fiancé cannot afford. I don't want one anyway. We have each other. I'll do anything he wants, and for a few months I believe I understand my father better, sympathize with his demand for respect. It makes sense in a way it never will again. This was a very long time ago; I am twenty-three, I *know* life, I'm certain about love, clear as glass. Then I hear the smallest of hisses. It's my vaso-vagal reflex again. I go down, separating myself from any future in surgery. This time, even I agree to stay in the doctor's lounge.

I learn later to pump calf muscles, shuffle my feet when standing still. I learn to mask my face, relaxing parents and patients, even though I'm never fully at ease myself. I become familiar with anatomic terms, Latinate shields doctors use to separate us-from-them. I'm never comfortable with this language of disguise, and revert to north Jersey slang every chance I get. This amuses my peers, vexes my professors. Junior year I'm told to read an x-ray, cold, in class, make a diagnosis. I get the disease right, but describe the lung masses as big balls. The professor is not pleased. *My dear, your father spent good money for your education. Couldn't you exert yourself to learn a little vocabulary?*

Dad isn't paying, I say. *I'm on scholarship.* And I am. First woman awarded this stipend, but I have to promise at the interview I won't marry until I've completed training. Easy to give my word at the time. I couldn't imagine myself married. I'd stopped longing for love after high school. But then he came, out of the blue, cerulean eyes, lashes so long they should be illegal, and a tongue that could sell the Brooklyn bridge to one hundred women at auction, each woman thinking she was the sole owner. I keep my maiden name until graduation, although we wed the end of my freshman year. I worry a lot about being found out; fear they'll take their money back.

Years after that first surgery, I grow a carapace, enter pediatric pathology. There's little night-call, the schedule's sane, eight to five or six, and I love looking through the microscope. Love it. Also, I can be home nights for my children. In medicine, as in life, there's a but. I have to perform autopsies on babies, teenagers, children, almost daily. I must enter the OR confident, during eye enucleations I get tissue for frozen sections, to confirm tumor. I witness brain surgeries, occasionally open heart procedures. I dissect limbs, severed legs and arms from car wrecks, from cancer, from the rare instance of physician stupidity. Still, I'm never able to watch someone else perform an autopsy without nausea and vertigo, and that atonal ring in my ear, cramping my heart to flutter. In a way this weakness is a relief, it means some part of me is still human.

Junior and senior years of medical school are more interesting, like my husband promised. But also harder: there's outpatient clinics, rounds on wards, scrubbing for surgeries, writing chart notes, learning new diseases, and days, months, of sleep deprivation. We numb, like we did as children learning scales with the piano teacher who drummed *every good boy deserves fun* over and over until auditory circuits closed and just the silk of ivory slipped beneath fingertips. I always wondered what good girls deserved, but now, there's neither time nor energy to worry equality. I can't listen long enough to a friend's problem, take a soaking bath, call home on Sunday, or hear Mozart's *Sinfonia Concertante* all the way through. Solitude, to repair what's unraveling, is only available in dreams. And nights now are too short for REM patterns to develop.

My graduation ceremony is June, 1968. Philadelphia, ninety-eight degrees, ninety-nine percent humidity. The street shimmers beneath the floor-length, black gabardine gown, further heating my seven-month-distended belly. There are minutes I almost dissolve in the small ancient church. We graduates are stored in the balcony, as deans drone on and the temperature rises. Our names are called; I am closer to mid-alphabet today. We descend a skinny, winding staircase I cannot see. I tap steps with my toe, clasp the shoulder of a friend ahead of me, play it by ear.

I smell him, my classmate, strong and sturdy, study partner for four years. In many ways I love this man. It's platonic. He and I play hooky together senior year, avoid the drear Philadelphia General neurology rotation, its patients with tertiary syphilis, intractable tremors, brains riddled by metastases. The deposited people who drool, soil themselves, sit swaddled in wheelchairs or beds. We go to the art museum, the zoo, catch a foreign flick, picnic along the Wissahickon, sunny afternoons.

My husband's last name is called. I cross the stage, take my sheepskin in Latin with my married name, assumed now in pride, that someone would actually marry me. I am tone deaf to feminist mantras.

At five p.m., the ceremony's complete. It's hotter. When my tassel's on the left, my parents insist on a photo shoot. They opposed medicine initially, no career for a woman. Who would marry a girl with that much education? They believed, common for the '60s, that after high school, or after college, for sure, I should marry. Even my sister, eight years my junior, is raised on Barbie pap. She complains to me now how desperately she wanted to be a doctor, all her life. *Why didn't you?* I ask once. *Women didn't do that then. Besides, I wanted to marry, have children.* And she did. Her marriage (which I admit, outlasts both of mine, even strung together) is strong and still sings with romance. Highschool sweethearts. *You would have made a great diagnostician*, I add. She says, *There were no role models back then, no good ones.*

But that hot, hot afternoon my parents are mysteriously proud. They pose us in squint-distorted shots until I say, "Shit. It's hot as friggin' hell in this. Hurry up. I need to take off this fucking gown."

Mother turns to Dad, *I told you we should've insisted on finishing school*, she says, in a stage whisper.

My first child's a daughter; healthy, whole. I have never known such happiness. Mother gives me talcum powder and a book, something for each end. Anne Morrow Lindbergh's *A Gift From the Sea*. In it, she writes that women are stronger because they have an internal cycle for more than half their lives. I'd think about this, about cyclicity, only I'm back on the medicine merry-go-round, praying the calliope doesn't stop, that it sounds sweet to my babygirl too. My belly collapses in after her birth, literally, and I take off two extra weeks. They "gave" me my vacation to have her. I do not want to return. I'm no longer interested in being a doctor. And it's not post-partum blues. But the interns course through our apartment, bearing gifts, promising a light schedule. My husband urges, reasonably, that I get this year behind me. I return to every-other-night call for the next ten months. That's officially thirty-six of every forty-eight hours, but in reality, it's forty, forty-two hour shifts. I get almost no sleep on-call. This is no different for any other intern. It's the *ten miles of snow in sub-zero, barefoot* that everyone romances their youth with when they think back. But it is cruel and stupid and toxic.

I grow thin enough to be diagnosed anorectic, but no one uses that term in '68. I lose my cycles completely. I don't miss a thing. Except laughter.

My medical school study partner has it worse, only I don't learn this for years. No one has time or energy to stay in touch during training, but his marriage fails during residency, a mutual friend confides at a national meeting much later. *One night he just walked off the Golden Gate Bridge.*

For me now, it's the psychedelic '70s; my husband and I are hippies at home, look respectable at work, although there is my underarm hair and a braid so long it sweeps my butt. I am still expected to defer, to look attractive, to keep up. Normal wives learn innovative lovemaking, try new casseroles. My husband and I protest the Vietnam War, sometimes with red-cross armbands, always with the children. They are photographed, in utero, in backpacks, small hands being held. We are a family striving for peace, in parades.

I also march with the children for the Equal Rights Amendment. I wear a white dress like suffragettes fifty years earlier. I think of Mother's frustrations with me, a tomboy climbing trees, coming to dinner muddy, never demure enough; how she wanted me to sing in a high register like she did. Me, a natural alto.

During residency I sometimes write notes on napkins in lectures, slip them into the white pockets of speakers. *Not every patient is female. Not all doctors are men.*

Everyone listens to the Beatles now, smokes dope, strums guitars. We have dinners and jam sessions at our home. My husband plays all string instruments, I can barely read music. He chords John Denver melodies each night after supper as I get the children ready for bed, clean up the dishes. I try to learn the banjo, half-try, but his playing's far better. His music is very seductive. We couldn't be happier.

After my first baby, I bring medical journals home, open them after she's asleep, after supper, fall unconscious in their pages. After the second birth, I still bring things home, pile them bedside, never open them. When our son arrives, I continue the professional charade, carry journals to the car, leave them neatly stacked for the next day.

Three children in four years; I am in trouble. A neurologist I haven't seen since internship enters a crowded elevator where I'm wedged, late in my third pregnancy, enormous. He raises his eyebrows, and his voice. *Don't you ever watch Carson, on the late show?* Everyone turns.

At work, brains take you only so far before a small high voice begins, in your head more than your ear, a mosquito before sunrise. It's difficult to distinguish from the chatter of lifesong: childbirth caws, pots banging for dinner, overhead pages, suckling babies, a home of music, and on-call phone messages. Like my partners, I do autopsies; learn to diagnose slides from surgical specimens; write PADs and FADs, preliminary and final diagnoses; describe the histology of the baby's organs, create a little biography. Short lives: prenatal history, what happened during the illness, what the therapy was, and what I found at post mortem. Then I do a review of the relevant literature.

One day, late in training, I find little corpses of beliefs I treasured stacked in my lap. I entered medicine to help people, to work in an exciting field, to remain independent. But even this "protected" residency includes some

weeks of twelve-hour days. Personal grooming stream-
lines, kindness pulls away like debriding charred skin.
Being patient or polite is alien as breathing oil.

It's in my denials, an emotional Braille that my husband, who is not blind, has no incentive to learn. My incessant fatigue wounds both of us. I stay awake to bathe
the children, rock them to sleep, read them stories. He's
a grown-up, he should understand. Hell, a few years back,
he did the same thing.

At work I stay strong, embrace too many parents as
they thunder *nooooo* down corridors after the news. It's
this continuous over-exposure to children's sicknesses
and dying schedules that depletes me. Life stretches tight
as a tympanic membrane. Pacing for a joke, an afternoon
window shopping, a crying jag, all gone. There are no
luxuries now beyond time.

Thirty years after graduation, mother's in a nursing
home, disabled with Parkinson's. She's frail and dying,
fades in and out of lucidity. When I can steal time from
my practice, from my second husband, from my children,
I visit. In return she musters her mind for the day. The
last coherent trip I wheel her out of the home, place her in
a rental car, drive to the ocean, thinking to revive, even
briefly, some of her early vigor.

I have questions.

How did you go on after Danny? I still ache for that baby
brother, forty-five years later, only five weeks of him. *Why
did you choose Dad against your mother's objections? Do
you have regrets? What would you do differently if you could
replay it?*

I want to know how she swallowed her pride at my dis-
missal, in the heady throes of adolescence, at thirteen,
so we might later reconcile. I'm having conflicts with
my own daughters now, whose visions wildly differ from
mine. *You raised us to think for ourselves,* they chorus. *Now
that we do, you can't even listen.* Does she have suggestions?

She answers so softly I have to lean down to hear. *I
made one big mistake, I should've had a career.*

Thinking the wind's sifted her words, or she's muddled again, I ask, *What did you say?*

I should have studied something. I could've earned...a living. Then, when he got mean, so awful. She shakes her head, or maybe it's the Parkinson's. *You have no idea what it was like, living with him, those years. Your father. No idea.*

I cradle her shoulders, wipe her tears. But I know, I want to say. Husband number two is no improvement over number one. I pray this is not heritable.

Mother flew to Denver after the birth of each baby. Our son was three months old before she came that last time. She said our household was too noisy, and chaotic. She said we needed privacy. I could've used her help. My husband worked late at the lab then, attended anti-war meetings most nights. Our babyboy got sick early in Mother's visit. It began with subtleties, a fussiness, he wouldn't nurse, he smelled funny, a sweet-sick scent I'd memorized on wards during my internship. When I held him normally to nurse or laid him down to change his diaper, he screamed. I could only cuddle him upright, against my chest, where he would quiet to a whimper. We take him to the ER. The on-call pediatrician checks him, twice. My husband and I watch him use his stethoscope, his otoscope. He checks ear canals, drums, heart, lungs, belly. He checks for hernias. *False alarm. Colic.*

By three a.m. a high fever erupts, by five, we're back at the hospital. I'm crazy with fear, meningitis, something about baby boys in my hands. They do a spinal tap, and a nurse, my partner's wife, our friend, walks me around and around while the tap's performed. She waits with us for results from the lab, my lab. I'm so scared, I cannot even hum a lullaby, although he's burning in my arms. I'm as distraught as every parent I've ever consoled, when pink goo leaks from his left ear to his shoulder, then to mine. A perforated eardrum. He recovers with antibiotics. Mother, who was at home with the girls, phones the airport, changes flights, leaves early. She was a superstitious woman.

At thirty, my residency is over. My marriage wobbles like a top at the end of a spin. I have three children, a handsome husband. The future should open like a ripe rose, mulched, petal-years, long before decay. But instead I crack, a pick fracturing ice. The day I disintegrate is sunny and warm, upstate New York, August. My sister is getting married. The people I see are not her guests. The bugs that crawl on me aren't the mosquitoes everyone else simply swats at dusk. My "people" make fun of my hips and belly, how slowly my mind works. They command me to change diapers. *You get shit patrol, because your eyes are brown. Because you are shit.* They probe me, engage in obscene acts. No one else hears them, luckily. Also, I can predict the future. It isn't pretty.

You'll lose your children for awhile, then you'll come back, only changed, you know, like throw-away plastic diapers.

The diagnosis is mumbo jumbo, *paranoid thought disorder, detachment from reality, verb salad, delusions, hallucinations. Schizophrenia.*

During my hospitalization an enormous abdominal hole, a through and through tunnel, burrows low in my belly, where my uterus completed all that begetting. I pass one hand through the front and clasp my other from behind, a secret handshake. This is decades before the cancer, but a strange prescience in the interminable morass of insanity. It takes months to convince them I'm sane, although I'm not. I need to get out, to get back to my children. It takes years to recover.

I bluster through the end of that marriage, the shaming divorce, anchor myself to my small children, to medicine. I puzzle over the microscope with its sea of cells, periwinkle borders, purple nuclei dividing, tumors needing names. I call surgeons, cook for, and read to, my children, teach residents and students, hang macramé on our windows, hang mobiles throughout the house, hug everyone, every chance I get. Like many mothers, I fret over childhood illnesses, behavior problems, their lost Dad.

Eventually, I try love again, buttressed by family and work.

Daylight hours are filled, overfilled, with congenital heart diseases, chromosome abnormalities, premature babies, a stream of childhood cancers, placentas. Slides, formaldehyde fumes, midnight frozen sections, speedy decisions race my mind. I run conferences, present papers at international meetings, with occasional applause for a minor point, the way Nana clapped when I made a good French knot, or Dad, when Mother sang pitch-perfect harmony with him.

It's decades and decades later when someone asks, *Would you do it all again?* And like so much after the fact, the answer is half notes, yes and no.

I create a list, my life is littered with lists: x-rays to review, teacher conferences to attend, ballet lessons for my daughters, preparation for grand rounds, groceries, cash for sitters, retrieving the children from soccer. *Be warned,* Nana said, *Advice is worth what you pay for it.* Here's mine, free, for anyone considering medicine: you will weigh each decision of your private life like a diagnosis, benign or malignant. You will use medical terminology, inappropriately, late at night, in a lover's arms. You will navigate your own emotional bed like a triage unit. You will enter therapy. You will be too busy. You will run eternally late.

You will ruin your easy laughter as you struggle to keep your word. You will quit: a husband, a field, a friend, but if you're very, very lucky, not your children.

In its favor, the title doctor guarantees last minute restaurant reservations. You will whittle your student loans down; you can take exotic educational vacations, tax deductible. But everyone will believe you have more money than Midas, and charge accordingly. You can stop at roadside accidents, legitimately, but you may spend precious minutes trying to convince crowds you really are a physician, especially if you're female, young, attractive. This will be exaggerated in foreign countries.

On a vacation in Sicily with my second husband once, a horrible motorcycle crash occurred just ahead of us. I knew no Italian; he cowered just thinking of blood or disease. Traffic was jammed. I jumped from the rental, ran to the scene, as the ambulance arrived. Medics, white-suited dancers, ran between the victim and the ambulance as blood spurted enthusiastically from his head and chest. I shouted *Doctore*, loud as I could, pointed to my chest, uncertain I'd be believed, or heard. Afraid I might be put in charge. I felt the man's wrist, his neck. No pulse. He was pale, young, unhelmeted; his chest did not move. The crowd stopped breathing; everyone froze except the white-clothed acrobats hanging a transfusion, pulling the IV extension higher, shouting orders to one another. They returned to the vehicle again and again, oxygen, a stethoscope, needles, alcohol. I watched for breath, for movement, repalpated his pulse, then left. Back at the Fiat, my husband started. *You didn't have gloves. There's AIDS everywhere today. Did you even consider me?* It's the beginning of our end, this harangue, and some part of me knows that. I sit and listen to him swear, to the sirens recede, impotent as anyone in the face of death. My weeping finally silences him.

Years later, after my radical hysterectomy, I *have* a huge hole in my belly. The cancer's out, but the husband rants in my hospital room, from fear no doubt, but it's so uncontrolled the nurses form an "evac" unit, remove him. I do not cry. I'm glad to be alive; glad to be cured, at least for the moment; glad to be.

So, if you enter medicine, you will fill, and overfill your days, mortgage your children's early years caring for others. You'll meet extraordinary men and women, yoked in service, some with God-complexes lacking compassion, but the majority are dedicated, an honor to work beside. I know, I was lucky most of my career.

A channeled whelk sits on my desk in honor of Anne Morrow Lindbergh. When the phone rings, I hope it's one of my children, or a close friend. It will not be the OR. If it's someone I don't care for, I hold the cool shell to my other ear. The opening coil emits a sound that might be middle C, if I had perfect pitch.

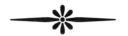

Namaste.